Veterinary Medical School Admission Requirements

nary Medical School Admission Requirements

2018 EDITION FOR 2019 MATRICULATION

ASSOCIATION OF AMERICAN VETERINARY MEDICAL COLLEGES

PURDUE UNIVERSITY PRESS | WEST LAFAYETTE, INDIANA

Please be aware that the admission requirements described in this book are subject to change by individual institutions without prior notice. Additionally, while VMCAS has made every effort to ensure the accuracy of the information contained in this book, VMCAS is not liable for any misrepresentations of a college's requirements. The provisions of this book do not constitute a contract between any applicant or student and the colleges of veterinary medicine.

COPYRIGHT © 2018 BY THE ASSOCIATION OF AMERICAN VETERINARY MEDICAL COLLEGES.
All rights reserved. Printed in the United States of America.

Compiled by the Association of American Veterinary Medical Colleges;
Tony Wynne, Editor, Director of Admissions and Recruitment Affairs

Paperback ISBN: 978-1-55753-817-8
ePub ISBN: 978-1-61249-531-6
ePDF ISBN: 978-1-61249-532-3
ISSN: 1089-6465

ACCEPTANCE DATE POLICY

In order to grant member schools enough time to complete their admissions processes and to give applicants enough time to consider all offers of admissions, no AAVMC Member Institution will require any applicant to make a decision about admission or financial aid before April 15 of each year. If April 15 falls on a Saturday or a Sunday, the date will be shifted to the following Monday.

To ensure applicants are awareness of this policy, each Member Institution will attach a copy of this policy to all admissions offer letters.

This policy does not apply to:

- Institutions outside the U.S. that do not participate in VMCAS
- Offers of admission for non-VMCAS applicants to institutions outside the U.S.
- Offers of admission for matriculation that is other than August or September

PROCEDURE

The Executive Director will investigate all complaints about alleged violations of this policy and report any findings to the chair of the Admissions and Recruitment Committee.

First Offense: If a Member Institution is found to be in violation of the policy, the Executive Director will send a Warning Letter to the Dean and Admissions Director of the institution and inform the Executive Committee of the Board of Directors.

Second and Subsequent Offenses: If a Member Institution is found to be in violation of this policy after a Warning Letter has been issued, the Executive Director and the chair of the Admissions and Recruitment Committee will report their findings to the Board of Directors and make a recommendation for additional penalties. Penalties may include monetary fines and exclusion from participation in VMCAS for a specified period of time.

Approved by the AAVMC Board of Directors
November 10, 2014

CONTENTS

FOREWORD

Congratulations on your decision to prepare for a career in veterinary medicine. Veterinary medicine is an exciting and rewarding career that provides a diverse array of options for contributing to the health of animals, people, and the planet.

Published annually by the Association of American Veterinary Medical Colleges (AAVMC), this *Veterinary Medical School Admission Requirements (VMSAR)* publication helps prospective students consider an important mix of factors when preparing for a veterinary medical education, including cost, financial aid, special programs, standardized tests, the AAVMC Veterinary Medical College Application Service (VMCAS), and the various colleges' and schools' residency admissions requirements.

Where to apply and attend will be one of your initial decisions, and it's an important one, but all of these American Veterinary Medical Association (AVMA)-accredited schools offer great programs. Each one can start you on a rewarding path filled with choices and opportunities. Animal clinical care is an important and popular option in veterinary medicine, but veterinarians also contribute to global health in many other ways, including through careers in public health, research, and specialty practice. You also can prepare yourself for scientific and administrative careers with pharmaceutical, nutrition, and biomedical health corporations, or work in state and federal government. Augmenting your professional degree with advanced graduate work can lead to faculty positions in higher education.

> Our profession offers many opportunities beyond the time-honored practice of providing clinical care in general practice.

Like other health professions, the pursuit and achievement of a veterinary medical education represents a substantial investment of time, effort, and financial resources. Cost-saving strategies include focusing on in-state veterinary medical schools or states that offer in-state tuition as part of special agreements with neighboring states. Other strategies include focusing on areas of greatest need, such as rural veterinary practice where loan repayment options might be available.

More information can be found on individual college and school websites or on the AAVMC website at www.aavmc.org. Prospective students also can contact the appropriate admissions office at each school or the VMCAS Student and Advisor Hotline, either by e-mail (vmcasinfo@vmcas.org) or by calling VMCAS at (617) 612-2884. The Veterinary Student Engagement System (VSES) is a useful tool as well.

Perhaps no other medical career provides such a broad base of biomedical training and leads to so many different areas of opportunity. The choices can seem overwhelming, but this guide is a great place to start, and step by step, your path will become clear, as it did for me. In my own case, a veterinary medical education led me to service as an officer in the United States Air Force, work in a mixed animal practice, in public health as an official with the U.S. Centers for Disease Control and Prevention, and now, as the chief executive officer of the AAVMC.

All of us at the AAVMC wish you luck and success as you prepare yourself for service in this extraordinary profession.

Dr. Andrew Maccabe
AAVMC Chief Executive Officer

ABOUT THE AAVMC

The Association of American Veterinary Medical Colleges (AAVMC) is a non-profit membership organization working to protect and improve the health and welfare of animals, people, and the environment by advancing academic veterinary medicine. The association was founded in 1966 by the deans of the then-existing eighteen colleges of veterinary medicine in the United States and three in Canada. During the 1970s and 1980s, AAVMC's membership expanded to include departments of veterinary science in colleges of agriculture, and in the 1990s to include divisions or departments of comparative medicine. In 2008, AAVMC began accepting non-accredited colleges and schools of veterinary medicine as affiliate members.

Today, AAVMC provides leadership for an academic veterinary medical community that includes all thirty colleges of veterinary medicine in the United States; nine departments of veterinary science; eight departments of comparative medicine; all five veterinary medical colleges in Canada; thirteen accredited colleges of veterinary medicine in Australia, Grenada, Ireland, Mexico, the Netherlands, New Zealand, St. Kitts, the United Kingdom, and six affiliate members.

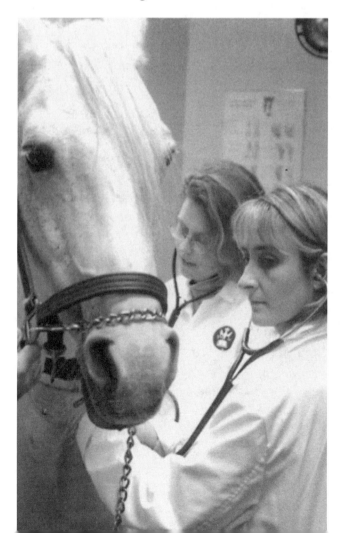

MISSION

AAVMC provides leadership for and promotes excellence in academic veterinary medicine to prepare the veterinary workforce with the scientific knowledge and skills required to meet societal needs through the protection of animal health, the relief of animal suffering, the conservation of animal resources, the promotion of public health, and the advancement of medical knowledge.

AAVMC pursues its mission by providing leadership in:

- Advocating on behalf of academic veterinary medicine;
- Serving as a catalyst and convener on issues of importance to academic veterinary medicine;
- Providing information, knowledge, and solutions to support members' work;
- Facilitating enrollment in veterinary medical schools and colleges; and
- Building global partnerships and coalitions to advance our collective goals.

STRATEGIC GOALS

1. Lead efforts to review, evaluate, and improve veterinary medical education in order to prepare graduates with the competencies needed to address societal needs.
2. Lead efforts to increase the amount of veterinary research conducted and the number of graduates entering research careers.
3. Lead efforts to recruit a student body aligned with the demands for veterinary expertise.
4. Lead efforts to increase the number of racially and/or ethnically underrepresented in veterinary medicine (URVM*) individuals throughout academic veterinary medicine.
5. Lead efforts to develop the next generation of leaders for academic veterinary medicine.
6. Strengthen AAVMC's capacity to better serve its members, partners, and other stakeholders in advancing the AAVMC mission.

*"URVMs are populations of individuals whose advancement in the veterinary medical profession have historically been disproportionately impacted by six specific aspects of diversity (gender, race, ethnicity, and geographic, socio-economic, and educational disadvantage) due to legal, cultural, or social climate impediments." *Definition of Underrepresented in Veterinary Medicine (URVM)*, approved by the AAVMC Board of Directors, July 20, 2008.

Left: A Tufts University Cummings School of Veterinary Medicine student checks out a horse with advice from her professor. Photo courtesy of Andy Cunningham of the Tufts University Cummings School of Veterinary Medicine.

VETERINARY MEDICINE: OPPORTUNITIES AND CHOICES

Veterinarians help animals and people live longer, healthier lives. They serve society through the protection of animal health and welfare, the prevention and relief of animal suffering, the conservation of animal resources, the promotion of public health, and the advancement of medical knowledge. The Doctor of Veterinary Medicine degree can lead to diverse career opportunities and different lifestyles from a solo mixed-animal practice in a rural area to a teaching or research position at an urban university, medical center, or industrial laboratory. The majority of veterinarians in the United States are in private clinical practice, although significant numbers are involved in preventive medicine, regulatory veterinary medicine, military veterinary medicine, laboratory animal medicine, research and development in industry, and teaching and research in a variety of basic science and clinical disciplines.

THE SPECTRUM OF OPPORTUNITIES IN VETERINARY MEDICINE

Veterinarians may choose to become specialists in a clinical area or to work with particular species. The first step on the path toward specialization is usually an internship.

1) FURTHER TRAINING

Internship

Internships are one-year programs in either small- or large-animal medicine and surgery. The most prestigious internship programs are at veterinary medical colleges or at very large private veterinary hospitals with board-certified veterinarians on staff. Since internships are usually at large referral centers, interns are exposed to a larger number of challenging cases than they would be likely to see in a smaller private practice.

Veterinary students in their senior year and veterinary graduates apply for internships through a matching program. Internship applicants and training hospitals rank each other in order of preference, and a computerized system matches each applicant with the highest-ranking teaching hospital that ranked the applicant. Academic performance in the veterinary professional curriculum, as well as recommendations from veterinary school faculty, is considered in the ranking of internship applicants.

Most veterinary interns in the United States receive a nominal salary, and their educational debts, if any, may be postponed in some governmentally subsidized loan programs. Veterinarians can sometimes command a higher starting salary in private practice after completion of an internship. Also, an internship is often the next step, after receiving the veterinary degree, toward residency and board certification.

Residency Training

Residency training is more specialized than an internship. Residency training programs are competitive and most require that the prospective residents complete an internship or equivalent private-practice experience prior to beginning the residency programs. Residency training is available in disciplines as varied as internal medicine, surgery, preventive medicine, behavior, toxicology, dentistry, and pathology.

The programs take two to three years to complete, depending on the nature of the specialty. Successful completion of a residency often is an important step toward attainment of board certification. Some residencies combine research and graduate study, leading to master's or PhD degrees.

Board Certification

Currently, there are twenty-two AVMA-recognized veterinary specialty organizations, comprising forty distinct specialties: anesthesiology, animal behavior, clinical pharmacology, dentistry, dermatology, emergency and critical care, internal medicine, laboratory animal medicine, microbiology, nutrition, ophthalmology, pathology, poultry medicine, private practice, preventive medicine, radiology, surgery, sports medicine and rehabilitation, theriogenology (reproduction), toxicology, and zoological medicine. Veterinarians may become board certified by completing rigorous postgraduate training, education, and examination requirements.

2) PRIVATE AND PUBLIC PRACTICE

The majority of veterinary graduates are engaged in private practice, either as an owner of a solo practice or, more likely, as a partner or associate in a group practice. Increasingly, veterinarians work together as a team, which allows a wider range of services to be provided.

Small-animal veterinarians focus their efforts primarily on dogs and cats but are seeing a growing number of other pets, including other small mammals, birds, reptiles, and fish.

Large-animal veterinarians often place their emphasis on horses, cattle, or pigs, and work both on a farm-call and an in-clinic basis. A mixed-animal veterinarian works with all types of domestic animals.

Public practice provides a variety of opportunities at the international, national, state, county, or city levels. There are exciting career opportunities for veterinarians in food safety, public health, the military, animal disease control, and research. Some veterinarians are employed by zoos and aquariums, wildlife conservation groups, game farms, or fisheries.

3) INDUSTRY

Veterinarians have many opportunities available to them in private industry, particularly in the fields of nutrition and pharmaceuticals. Assisting in the development of new products in the animal industry, conducting research for pharmaceutical companies, diagnosing disease and drug effects as pathologists, or safeguarding the health of laboratory animal colonies are all interesting career possibilities.

4) CONCLUSION

By the very nature of the comparative medical education that veterinarians receive, the many species of animals they care for and work for, and the wide variety of clientele served, the opportunities available to today's veterinarian are abundant.

INFORMATION ABOUT STANDARDIZED TESTS

Most veterinary medical colleges require one or more standardized tests: the Graduate Record Examination (GRE) or the Medical College Admission Test (MCAT). For further information regarding test dates and registration procedures, contact the testing agencies listed below:

GRE Graduate Record Examinations
P.O. Box 6000
Princeton, NJ 08541-6000
(609) 771-7670 (Princeton, NJ)
also: (510) 654-1200 (Oakland, CA)
www.gre.org
Individual school codes: see GRE booklet

MCAT Medical College Admission Test
MCAT Program Office
P.O. Box 4056
Iowa City, IA 52243-4056
(319) 337-1357
www.aamc.org/students/applying/mcat

TOEFL Test of English as a Foreign Language
TOEFL/TSE Services
P.O. Box 6151
Princeton, NJ 08541-6151
(609) 771-7100
www.toefl.org

AAVMC MEMBER INSTITUTIONS AND THE ROLE OF ACCREDITATION

Veterinary Schools join the AAVMC as institutional or affiliate members. A key difference between these two membership categories is whether a college/school of veterinary medicine is accredited by the Council on Education (COE). Only COE-accredited colleges of veterinary medicine may join AAVMC as an institutional (voting) member. Colleges of veterinary medicine that are not COE-accredited may join AAVMC as an affiliate member (non-voting) only. Several of AAVMC's affiliate members (non-COE–accredited institutions) have entered into agreements with AAVMC institutional members for clinical training. It is important for prospective veterinary students to know the different implications of attending and/or graduating from COE-accredited vs. non-COE–accredited colleges of veterinary medicine as it pertains to educational options and eventually seeking and obtaining a license to practice veterinary medicine. AAVMC encourages its affiliate members to become COE-accredited.

ACCREDITATION

The COE accredits DVM or equivalent educational programs. Accreditation through the COE assures that minimum standards in veterinary medical education are met by accredited colleges of veterinary medicine and that students enrolled in these colleges receive an education that will prepare them for entry-level positions in the profession. In the United States, graduation from a COE-accredited college of veterinary medicine is an important prerequisite for application for licensure. Internationally, some veterinary schools have chosen to seek COE accreditation in addition to accreditation by the competent authority in their own regions. COE accreditation of international veterinary schools provides assurance that those programs of education meet the same standards as other similarly accredited schools.

Additionally, COE accreditation assures:
- Prospective students that they will meet a competency threshold for entry into practice, including eligibility for professional credentialing and/or licensure;
- Employers that graduates have achieved specified learning goals and are prepared to begin professional practice;
- Faculty, deans, and administrators that their programs measure satisfactorily against national standards and their own stated missions and goals;

- The public that public health and safety concerns are being addressed; and
- The veterinary profession that the science and art of veterinary medicine are being advanced through contemporary curricula.

*Source: The source for this information and a site recommended for obtaining additional information is as follows: https://www.avma.org/ProfessionalDevelopment/Education/Accreditation/Colleges/Pages/about-accred.aspx

LICENSURE

Licensure in the United States

In the United States, requirements for licensure are set by individual state regulatory boards. The North American Veterinary Licensing Exam (NAVLE) and any additional state exams must be taken by a graduate to become eligible for state licensure. The NAVLE, which is administered by the International Council for Veterinary Assessment (ICVA), fulfills a core requirement for licensure to practice veterinary medicine in all jurisdictions in the United States and Canada. Mexico does not require NAVLE. In addition to the NAVLE, state regulatory boards will have other licensure requirements, which may include state-specific examinations.

To be eligible to take the NAVLE, applicants must have graduated from either a COE-accredited college of veterinary medicine or a non-COE–accredited college (see following details).

Applicants who graduated from a non-COE–accredited college must also have a certification of eligibility, which can come from one of two sources: the Educational Commission for Foreign Veterinary Graduates (ECFVG) Certification Program (www.avma.org /professionaldevelopment/education/foreign/pages/default.aspx) or the Program for the Assessment of Veterinary Education Equivalence (PAVE) (www.aavsb.org/PAVE).

All state regulatory boards accept the ECFVG certification, administered through the American Veterinary Medical Association (AVMA), as meeting in full or in part the educational prerequisite for licensure eligibility. At this time, twenty-eight state regulatory boards also accept PAVE certification, which is administered through the American Association of Veterinary State Boards (AAVSB).

It is important to note that prerequisites for licensure eligibility and requirements for licensure vary amongst state regulatory boards and are subject to periodic modification.

Licensure Outside the United States

Mutual recognition arrangements apply to jurisdictions where there are COE-accredited schools. These specify that graduates of COE-accredited schools in the United States and Canada are permitted to obtain licensure to practice under terms no less favorable than graduates of schools accredited by the competent authority in that jurisdiction.

DECIDING WHERE TO APPLY

There are several factors, as well as the issue of accreditation, that an applicant must consider in identifying school(s) to submit an application for admissions. In addition to licensure issues, there may be economic, educational options, or other differences that students should consider in making decisions on where to apply. This book is intended to provide important information about AAVMC members to assist in informed decision-making for students considering applying to one or more veterinary colleges.

PRE-VETERINARY PROFILE: ME'NISHA JONES

Current School Name
University of Central Florida

What type of veterinary medicine are you interested in pursuing, and why?
As of right now, I want to go into small animal medicine, but I also want to be a well-rounded vet who can help any animal.

What is/was your major during undergraduate school?
Psychology with a pre-veterinary track.

What are your short-term and long-term goals?
My short-term goals are to finish classes and apply to vet school, and my long-term goal is to graduate from vet school.

What are you doing as an applicant/pre-vet to prepare for veterinary school?
I am continuing to take courses that are prerequisites for graduate school, and I am getting jobs in the vet field to keep my dream alive.

What extracurricular activities are you involved in currently?
I was involved in Pre-Vet Society; I was President of First Knights, an organization dedicated to first-generation students; and I was involved SISTUHS Incorporated, dedicated to community service in the community. I was also a brother in the prestigious Alpha Kappa Psi Business Fraternity, and I served as Progressive Black Men's Miss Emerald for the 2016–2017 school year.

How old were you when you first became interested in being a veterinarian?
I was in tenth grade when I watched the sad ASPCA commercial that convinced me to make a difference in the lives of animals and to give them a voice.

Please describe your various experiences in preparation for applying to veterinary school.
I have already accepted my fate that I will be a nontraditional student, which can discourage some students. I have come to terms with the fact that, regardless of how long it takes me to get to vet school, as long as I keep my eye on the prize, nothing will stop me from my ultimate goal.

What characteristics are you looking for in a veterinary school?
II am looking for a challenging, helping vet school that will prepare me for situations that might occur in the real world of practice.

What advice do you have for other pre-veterinary students?
I advise students to never give up. Everyone's journey will not be the same, so don't focus on how everyone else is getting there—focus on what you have to do to get there. With determination and hard work, you can accomplish whatever you put your mind to.

GEOGRAPHICAL LISTING OF AAVMC INSTITUTIONAL (COE ACCREDITED) VETERINARY SCHOOLS AND DIRECTORY OF ADMISSIONS OFFICES

Atlantic Veterinary College at the
  University of Prince Edward
  Island (CANADA)
Registrar's Office
550 University Avenue
Charlottetown PEI C1A 4P3
Canada

Auburn University (USA)
Office for Academic Affairs
College of Veterinary Medicine
217 Goodwin/Overton
Auburn, AL 36849-5536

Colorado State University (USA)
College of Veterinary Medicine and
  Biomedical Sciences
1601 Campus Delivery – Office of
  the Dean
Fort Collins, CO 80523-1601

Cornell University (USA)
Office of Student & Academic Services
College of Veterinary Medicine
S2-009 Schurman Hall
Ithaca, NY 14853-6401

Iowa State University (USA)
Office of Admissions
College of Veterinary Medicine
2270 Veterinary Medicine
P.O. Box 3020
Ames, IA 50010-3020

Kansas State University (USA)
Office of Admissions
College of Veterinary Medicine
101 Trotter Hall
Manhattan, KS 66506-5601

Lincoln Memorial University (USA)
College of Veterinary Medicine
6965 Cumberland Gap Pkway
Harrogate, TN 37752

Louisiana State University (USA)
Office of Student and Academic Affairs
School of Veterinary Medicine
Skip Bertman Drive
Baton Rouge, LA 70803

Massey University Veterinary School
  (AUSTRALIA)
International Student Affairs
Undergraduate Office
IVABS
Private Bag 11-222
Palmerston North 4442
New Zealand

Michigan State University (USA)
Office of Admissions
College of Veterinary Medicine
784 Wilson Road
F-110 Veterinary Medical Center
East Lansing, MI 48824

Midwestern University (USA)
College of Veterinary Medicine
19555 North 59th Avenue
Glendale, AZ 85308

Mississippi State University (USA)
Office of Student Admissions
College of Veterinary Medicine
P.O. Box 6100
Mississippi State, MS 39762

Murdoch University
  (AUSTRALIA)
Murdoch International
South Street
Murdoch 6150
Western Australia

North Carolina State University (USA)
Student Services Office
College of Veterinary Medicine
1060 William Moore Drive, Box 8401
Raleigh, NC 27607

The Ohio State University (USA)
Office of Student Affairs
College of Veterinary Medicine
Suite 127 Veterinary Medicine
  Academic Building
1900 Coffey Road
Columbus, OH 43210-1089

Oklahoma State University (USA)
Office of Admissions
112 McElroy Hall
Center for Veterinary Health
  Sciences
College of Veterinary Medicine
Stillwater, OK 74078-2003

Oregon State University (USA)
Office of the Dean
Attention: Admissions
College of Veterinary Medicine
200 Magruder Hall
Corvallis, OR 97331-4801

Purdue University (USA)
Student Services Center
College of Veterinary Medicine
625 Harrison Street
West Lafayette, IN 47907-2026

Ross University School of Veterinary
  Medicine (ST. KITTS)
Office of Admissions
630 US HWY 1
North Brunswick, NJ 08902

Royal Veterinary College
  (UNITED KINGDOM)
Head of Admissions
Royal College Street
London NW1 0TU
United Kingdom

St. George's University
  (GRENADA)
Office of Admission
c/o The North American
  Correspondent
University Support Services, LLC
3500 Sunrise Highway
Building 300
Great River, NY 11739

Texas A & M University (USA)
Office of the Dean
College of Veterinary Medicine
  & Biomedical Sciences
College Station, TX 77843-4461

Tufts University (USA)
Office of Admissions
Cummings School of Veterinary
  Medicine
200 Westboro Road
North Grafton, MA 01536

Tuskegee University (USA)
Office of Admissions and
  Recruitment
School of Veterinary Medicine
100 Dr. Frederick Patterson Hall
Tuskegee, AL 36088

Universidad Nacional Autónoma
  de México (MEXICO)
Office of Undergraduate
  Studies (Division de Estudios
  Profesionales)
College of Veterinary Medicine
  (FMVZ)
Av. Universidad 3000
Circuito Interior
Delegacion Coyoacan
Mexico D.F. 04510

Université de Montréal (CANADA)
Service des Admissions
C.P. 6205
Succursale Centre-Ville
Montréal Québec H3C 3T5 Canada

University of Calgary (CANADA)
Admissions Office
Faculty of Veterinary Medicine
TRW 2D03
3280 Hospital Drive NW
Calgary, AB T2N 4Z6

University of California (USA)
School of Veterinary Medicine
Office of the Dean-Student
  Programs
One Shields Avenue
Davis, CA 95616

University College Dublin
  (IRELAND)
Veterinary Medicine Applications
UCD Admissions Office
Tierney Building
Belfield, Dublin 4
Ireland

University of Edinburgh
  (UNITED KINGDOM)
Admissions Office
Royal (Dick) School of Veterinary
  Studies
Easter Bush Veterinary Centre
Roslin EH25 9RG
Scotland

University of Florida (USA)
Admissions Office
College of Veterinary Medicine
P.O. Box 100125
Gainesville, FL 32610-0125

The University of Georgia (USA)
Admissions Department
Office for Academic Affairs
College of Veterinary Medicine
Athens, GA 30602-7372

University of Glasgow
  (UNITED KINGDOM)
Director of Admissions & Student
  Services Manager
College of Medicine, Veterinary and
  Life Sciences
School of Veterinary Medicine
  Undergraduate School
464 Bearsden Road
Glasgow G61 1QH

University of Guelph (CANADA)
Admissions Services
University Centre, Level 3
Guelph Ontario N 1G 2W 1
Canada

University of Illinois (USA)
College of Veterinary Medicine
Office of Academic and Student
  Affairs
2001 South Lincoln Avenue,
  Room 2271g
Urbana, IL 61802

University of Melbourne
  (AUSTRALIA)
Faculty of Veterinary Science
Corner Park Drive and
  Flemington Road
Parkville
Melbourne 3010
Victoria Australia

University of Minnesota (USA)
Office of Academic and Student Affairs
College of Veterinary Medicine
108 Pomeroy Center
1964 Fitch Ave.
St. Paul, MN 55108

University of Missouri-Columbia
  (USA)
Office of Academic Affairs
College of Veterinary Medicine
W203 Veterinary Medicine Building
Columbia, MO 65211

University of Pennsylvania (USA)
Admissions Office
School of Veterinary Medicine
3800 Spruce Street
Philadelphia, PA 19104-6044

The University of Queensland–
  Gatton Campus (AUSTRALIA)
School of Veterinary Science
Gatton, 4343
Queensland, Australia

University of Saskatchewan (CANADA)
Admissions Office
Western College of Veterinary Medicine
52 Campus Drive
Saskatoon Saskatchewan S7N 5B4
Canada

Sydney School of Veterinary Science (AUSTRALIA)
Faculty of Veterinary Science
Sydney, NSW 2006
Australia

University of Tennessee (USA)
Admissions Office
College of Veterinary Medicine
2407 River Drive
Room A-104-C
Knoxville, TN 37996-4550

University of Wisconsin-Madison (USA)
Office of Academic Affairs
School of Veterinary Medicine
2015 Linden Drive
Madison, WI 53706-1102

Utrecht University (NETHERLANDS)
Office for International Cooperation
Faculty of Veterinary Medicine
Yalelaan 1
3584 CL Utrecht
The Netherlands

VetAgro Sup (FRANCE)
1, avenue Bourgelat
69280 Marcy l'Etoile
France

Virginia-Maryland College of Veterinary Medicine (USA)
Admissions Coordinator
Blacksburg, VA 24061

Washington State University (USA)
Office of Student Services
College of Veterinary Medicine
100 Grimes Way
P.O. Box 647012
Pullman, WA 99164-7012

Western University of Health Sciences (USA)
Office of Admissions
College of Veterinary Medicine
309 East 2nd Street
Pomona, CA 91766-1854

GEOGRAPHICAL LISTING OF AAVMC AFFILIATE (NON-COE ACCREDITED) VETERINARY SCHOOLS AND DIRECTORY OF ADMISSIONS OFFICES

University of Adelaide
  (AUSTRALIA)
The School of Animal and
  Veterinary Science
Roseworthy Campus
Roseworthy SA 5371
Australia

Central Luzon State University
  (PHILIPPINES)
Science City of Munoz
Nueva Ecija 3120
Philippines

University of Copenhagen
  (DENMARK)
Office for International Cooperation
Faculty of Health and Medicine
Blegdamsvej 3B
DK-2200 Copenhagen N
Denmark

Seoul National University
  (SOUTH KOREA)
1 Gwanak-ro
Gwanak-gu, Seoul
South Korea

St. Matthew's University
  (WEST INDIES)
Office of Admissions
12124 High Tech Avenue,
Suite 350
Orlando, Fl 32817

United Arab Emirates University
  (UNITED ARAB EMIRATES)
  PO Box 15551 Al-Ain, United
  Arab Emirates

University of Tokyo (JAPAN)
1-1-1, Yayoi, Bunkyo-Ku
Tokyo 113-8657, Japan

University of Veterinary and Animal
  Sciences - UVAS (PAKISTAN)
Syed Abdul Qadir Jillani (Out Fall)
  Road, Lahore - Pakistan

LISTING OF CONTRACTING STATES AND PROVINCES

Six Canadian provinces and 19 states in the United States have a veterinary school contract with one or more schools to provide access to veterinary medical education for their residents. The state or province, working through the contracting agency, usually agrees to pay a fee to help cover the cost of education for a certain number of places in each entering class. Residents from the contract states then compete with each other for those positions.

Some states contract with more than one school. For example, Arkansas contracts with 5 veterinary schools, and North Dakota contracts with 6 schools. Connecticut, Rhode Island, Vermont, Nebraska, and the District of Columbia presently have no contracts, so all candidates from these places apply as nonresidents to veterinary schools of their choice.

The educational agreements between contracting agencies and veterinary schools differ. Under some contract arrangements, students pay in-state tuition; in others, they pay nonresident tuition. Some contract states require students to repay all or part of the subsidy that the state provided; others require veterinary graduates to return to practice in the state for a period of time. Applicants should be aware of their obligation to the state before agreeing to participate in a contract program.

Following is a list of states and provinces that have educational agreements with schools of veterinary medicine.

UNITED STATES

ARIZONA

Contracts through WICHE* with Colorado State University, Oregon State University, and Washington State University.

ARKANSAS

Contracts through the SREB** with Louisiana State University, University of Missouri, and Oklahoma State University. Contracts not all completed at time of printing; may be some changes.

DELAWARE

Contracts with Oklahoma State University and the University of Georgia.

HAWAII

Contracts through WICHE* with Colorado State University, Oregon State University, and Washington State University.

IDAHO

Contracts with Washington State University.

KENTUCKY

Contracts with Auburn University and Tuskegee University.

MONTANA

Contracts with Washington State University. Contracts through WICHE* with Colorado State University, Oregon State University, and Washington State University.

NEBRASKA

Formal education alliance with Iowa State University allows students admitted into the 2+2 program with the University of Nebraska-Lincoln to pay resident tuition for all 4 years.

NEVADA

Contracts through WICHE* with Colorado State University, Oregon State University, and Washington State University.

NEW MEXICO

Contracts through WICHE* with Colorado State University, Oregon State University, and Washington State University.

NORTH DAKOTA

Contracts with Iowa State University, University of Minnesota, and Kansas State University. Contracts through WICHE* with Colorado State University, Oregon State University, and Washington State University.

SOUTH CAROLINA

Contracts with University of Georgia, Mississippi State University, and Tuskegee University.

SOUTH DAKOTA

Reciprocity with University of Minnesota. Contracts with Iowa State University.

UTAH

Contracts with Washington State University.

---

* WICHE = Western Interstate Commission for Higher Education (offices in Boulder, Colorado)
**SREB = Southern Regional Educational Board

WEST VIRGINIA

Contracts with Mississippi State University and Virginia-Maryland College of Veterinary Medicine.

WYOMING

Contracts through WICHE* with Colorado State University, Oregon State University, and Washington State University.

CANADA

ALBERTA

Contracts with University of Calgary.

BRITISH COLUMBIA

Contracts with University of Saskatchewan.

MANITOBA

Contracts with University of Saskatchewan.

NEW BRUNSWICK

Contracts with Atlantic Veterinary College at the University of Prince Edward Island and Université de Montréal.

NEWFOUNDLAND

Contracts with Atlantic Veterinary College at the University of Prince Edward Island.

NOVA SCOTIA

Contracts with Atlantic Veterinary College at the University of Prince Edward Island.

* WICHE = Western Interstate Commission for Higher Education (offices in Boulder, Colorado)

PROGRAMS FOR MULTICULTURAL OR DISADVANTAGED STUDENTS

The Association of American Veterinary Medical Colleges affirms the value of diversity within the veterinary medical profession. The membership is committed to incorporating that belief into their actions by advocating for the recruitment and retention of underrepresented persons as students and faculty, and ultimately fostering their success in the profession of veterinary medicine. The Association believes that through these actions, society and the profession will be well served.

Many schools have programs designed to facilitate entry into, and retention by, veterinary programs nationwide. These programs are directed at several levels, from high-school students to the student who has already been accepted by a veterinary college. Most of these programs will accept students from every state, regardless of the school(s) to which an individual might eventually apply or attend.

Following is an alphabetical list of schools by state and a short explanation of their programs:

UNIVERSITY OF CALIFORNIA

Program: Summer Enrichment Program

Description: A 6-week summer program. The purpose of this program is to increase the academic preparedness of disadvantaged students through science-based learning skills development, clinical education, individual advising, and student development.

Eligibility: Educationally and/or economically disadvantaged. Must have completed at least one year of college with a minimum science GPA of 2.8 and demonstrated interest in veterinary medicine.

Program dates: July–August.

Contact: Office of the Dean–Student Programs, School of Veterinary Medicine, University of California, One Shields Avenue, Davis CA 95616; telephone: (530) 752-1383.

Sponsorship: School of Veterinary Medicine, University of California-Davis.

COLORADO STATE UNIVERSITY

Program: Vet Prep

Description: A one-year academic program that serves as a bridge to the Doctor of Veterinary (DVM) program for disadvantaged (cultural, social, economic) applicants who ranked high but were not admitted. Limited to 10 students who upon successful completion are guaranteed admission to the DVM program. Candidates are selected from the current regular admissions applicant pool and do not directly apply to the Vet Prep program.

Eligibility: Disadvantaged students.

Contact: College of Veterinary Medicine and Biomedical Sciences, W102 Anatomy, Colorado State University, Fort Collins CO 80523; telephone: (970) 491-7051; email: DVMAdmissions@colostate.edu.

Sponsorship: College of Veterinary Medicine and Biomedical Sciences, Colorado State University.

CORNELL UNIVERSITY

Program: State University of New York Graduate Underrepresented Minority Fellowships

Description: All matriculating underrepresented minorities are eligible (not restricted by state residency).

Contact: Director of Student Financial Planning, Office of Student & Academic Services, College of Veterinary Medicine, Cornell University, S2-009 Schurman Hall, Ithaca NY 14853-6401; telephone: (607) 253-3766; website: www.vet.cornell.edu/financialaid.

MICHIGAN STATE UNIVERSITY

Program: Enrichment Summer Program (ESP)

Description: The ESP, sponsored by the Michigan State University College of Veterinary Medicine with support of an endowment, provides academic advancement and career knowledge for undergraduate students interested in veterinary medicine. There is no fee to participate in this program.

Eligibility: The program is open to undergraduate students who have selected veterinary medicine as a career choice and plan to apply to a professional program. It focuses on developing well-qualified prospective students from disadvantaged backgrounds. Consideration is given to residents of Michigan who have a cumulative GPA of 3.0 or higher.

Program dates: Early June through late June.

How Do I Apply: The application opens November 1 each year and closes in late January. For more information, visit cvm.msu.edu/esp.

Contact: The Office of Diversity and Inclusion, College of Veterinary Medicine, 784 Wilson Road, F-113 B, Veterinary Medical Center, Michigan State University, East Lansing, MI 48824; telephone: (517) 355-6521; email: cvm.Diversity@cvm.msu.edu.

MISSISSIPPI STATE UNIVERSITY

Program: Board of Trustees of State Institutions of Higher Learning Veterinary Medicine Minority Loan/Scholarship Program

Description: A financial assistance program for Mississippi residents who are underrepresented minorities. The loan to service obligation is one year for each year of scholarship assistance, not to exceed four years.

Contact: Susan Eckels, Program Administrator, Mississippi Institutions of Higher Learning, 3825 Ridgewood Road, Jackson MS 39211-6453; telephone: (800) 327-2980.

Program: Vet Camp

Description: MSU-CVM has been offering Veterinary Camp since 2011. Modeled after the first and second year student experience, our curriculum is heavily hands-on and is taught by our own faculty, with DVM students serving as counselors and leaders. After that first year, the camp grew in the number of students we could serve, the number and types of camps we offered, and the labs and activities we provided. We are proud of the 100% satisfaction rate and willingness to recommend our camp reported by campers, parents, and our own faculty. We love sharing the veterinary profession with young people.

Program: VetAspire

Description: VetAspire is an exciting program designed for students to spend the day at Mississippi State University's College of Veterinary Medicine. Each month, five students will have the opportunity to participate in clinics, lectures, and hands-on activities. The goal of this program is to expose students to the field of veterinary medicine in hopes that they will choose it as a career path. Students will also get to see the real-world impact of math, science, and communications training.

Eligibility: Open to 11th and 12th grade high school students and college freshmen. Must be educationally, economically, and/or socially disadvantaged. All students (11th grade-college senior) will be considered, but priority will be given to students who meet the above criteria.

NORTH CAROLINA STATE UNIVERSITY

Program: UNC Campus Scholarship Program—Graduate Student Component

Description: UNC General Administration funds this program. Eligibility is limited to new or continuing full-time doctoral students who have financial need and who are residents of North Carolina as of the be-

ginning of the award period (as determined under the *Manual to Assist the Public Higher Education Institutions of N.C. in the Matter of Student Resident Classification for Tuition Purposes*). Individuals who have been accepted to a master's degree program in a department offering the doctoral degree and who intend, and will be eligible, to pursue doctoral studies at NC State after completion of the requirements for the master's degree are also eligible. The program provides up to $3,000 annually for North Carolina residents.

Contact: Director of Diversity Affairs, College of Veterinary Medicine, North Carolina State University, 1060 William Moore Drive, Box 8401, Raleigh, NC 27607; telephone: (919) 513-6262; website: www.cvm.ncsu.edu.

Program: Diversity Graduate Assistant Grant

Description: Funded by the North Carolina State University Graduate School, recipients must be full-time, new or continuing students pursuing master's and doctoral degrees at North Carolina State University. The program provides up to $3,000 annually. Both resident and nonresident students are eligible to apply.

Contact: Director of Diversity Affairs, College of Veterinary Medicine, North Carolina State University, 1060 William Moore Drive, Box 8401, Raleigh, NC 27607; telephone: (919) 513-6262; website: www.cvm.ncsu.edu.

Note: North Carolina residents are encouraged to apply for both programs. However, the annual maximum award for these grant programs is a combined $3,000 (with an option of $500 in additional support for study in the summer). The grant is awarded on an annual basis. Awardees must reapply each year.

THE OHIO STATE UNIVERSITY

Program: Buckeye Veterinary Camp

Description: In this summer residential camp, high school students will learn more about veterinary school and the profession.

Eligibility: Scholarships are available for those who qualify.

Program dates: Application typically opens in September-January. Dates of the camp are at the end of June.

Sponsorship: the State of Ohio and The Ohio State University.

Program: Summer Research Opportunities Program (SROP)

Description: The Summer Research Opportunities Program (SROP) at Ohio State is designed to help historically underrepresented students explore opportunities for graduate study and academic careers. Over the course of eight weeks during the summer, Ohio State SROP participants will conduct research with a faculty mentor on a topic of mutual interest, and participate in activities crucial to preparation for graduate school, including workshops on research skills, seminars on topics related to graduate education, and professional development events. At the end of the summer program, participants present their research at a campus summary conference and a regional conference.

Eligibility: All historically underrepresented undergraduates who are U.S. citizens and who meet the criteria listed in the qualifications section below are eligible to participate in the program. The selection process targets groups underrepresented in graduate education. Priority is given to those students who have not participated in SROP previously.

Contact: Graduate Student Recruitment, 614-247-6377, gradrecruit@osu.edu. Website: https://gradsch.osu.edu /research/summer-research-opportunities-program. SROP is overseen by the Big Ten Academic Alliance.

PURDUE UNIVERSITY

Program: Access to Animal-Related Careers (A²RC)

Description: A²RC is a two-week, residential program offering hands-on experiences in multiple areas of veterinary medicine including swine production medicine, small animal medicine, and equine medicine. Also included are sessions on several specialty areas such as cardiology, emergency and critical care medicine, and radiology. The program is designed to expose participants to life as a first year DVM student. Mock admissions interviews are conducted and participants are given individual feedback.

Eligibility: A²RC is targeted to 2nd and 3rd year underrepresented minority undergraduate students at partner institutions enrolled in pre-veterinary studies.

Program dates: May 13-26, 2018.

Contact: Office for Diversity and Inclusion (765-496-1940), website: https://www.vet.purdue.edu/diversity

UNIVERSITY OF TENNESSEE

Program: Veterinary Summer Experience for Tennessee High School Students

Description: The College of Veterinary Medicine offers an eight-week program that provides high school students an opportunity to gain experience working with veterinarians at a veterinary practice in their home towns for seven weeks during the summer. During the eighth week of this summer experience, students will be guests of the College of Veterinary Medicine on the campus of The University of Ten-

nessee in Knoxville. Students will attend clinical rotations in the Equine, Farm Animal, Small Animal, and Avian and Exotic Animal (including zoo medicine) Hospitals in the Veterinary Medical Center. Students will also attend special educational functions related to veterinary medicine.

Eligibility: To qualify for this summer program, a student must be a Tennessee resident and be at least 16 years of age by June 1, be enrolled as a senior or junior in a Tennessee high school, and have earned a minimum 3.0 high school GPA. Applicants must also have an interest in veterinary medicine as a potential career. Preference will be given to applicants who will contribute greatly to the diversity of the summer program and, potentially, to the veterinary profession. Students receive a financial stipend for satisfactory performance in the eight-week program.

Program dates: Summer.

Contact: Dr. William Hill, The University of Tennessee, College of Veterinary Medicine, 2431 Joe Johnson Drive, 339 Ellington Plant Science, Knoxville TN 37996, telephone: (865) 974-5770. E-mail: wahill@utk.edu.

UNIVERSITY OF MINNESOTA

Program: Veterinary Leadership in Early Admissions for Diversity (VetLEAD)

Description: VetLEAD creates a pathway into the DVM program for high-ability students at underrepresented serving partner schools, including Florida Agricultural and Mechanical University (FAMU).

Eligibility: Any high-achieving student enrolled in the Animal Science program at FAMU may apply for an early admissions decision at the end of their sophomore year of undergraduate studies. Eligible students have past experience working or volunteering in a veterinary related setting, a FAMU cumulative GPA of 3.4 with coursework consistent with required prerequisite courses, and strong letters of references.

Contact: Karen Nelson, Director of Admissions, dvminfo@umn.edu

TUSKEGEE UNIVERSITY

Program: Tuskegee University Summer Enrichment and Reinforcement Program (SERP)

Description: This is an exclusive program available only to accepted first year students. The SERP five-week program is a great introduction to the highly anticipated veterinary curriculum. It is an opportunity to strengthen the student's performance, surrounded by others who share their passion for animals, health, and science. The program focuses on the following key areas: critical thinking, analysis and application of clinical information, and learning strategies.

Eligibility: Participation is restricted to first year students accepted to the Tuskegee University College of Veterinary Medicine.

Program dates: May 29 through June 29, 2018

Contact: Kheri Spence, Assistant Director for Student Success/Counselor, College of Veterinary Medicine, Patterson Hall, 1200 W. Old Montgomery Road, Tuskegee Institute, Al 36088, telephone (334) 724-4247, email: kspence@tuskegee.edu.

Program: Veterinary Science Training, Education and Preparation Institute (Vet STEP)

Description: A residential program designed to introduce underrepresented minority high school students to exciting careers in veterinary medicine. Students spend a week on the campus of Tuskegee University learning about what it takes to be a veterinarian while attending stimulating academic classes. The all inclusive tuition for Vet STEP is $500.00.

Eligibility: Participation in Vet STEP I is restricted to high school students in 9th and 10th grade. Participation in Vet STEP II is restricted to high school students in 11th and 12th grade.

Contact: LaTia McCurdy, Coordinator of Veterinary Recruitment, Tuskegee University College of Veterinary Medicine, Patterson Hall, 1200 W. Montgomery Road, Tuskegee Institute, Al 36088. Telephone: (334) 727-8309, email: lmccurdy@tuskegee.edu.

VIRGINIA-MARYLAND COLLEGE OF VETERINARY MEDICINE

Program: VetTRAC Summer Program

Description: A weeklong program, VetTRAC aims to teach, inspire, mentor, engage, excite, and enlighten students from underrepresented populations with respect to the field of veterinary medicine to promote diversity and inclusion within the VA-MD College of Veterinary Medicine and the veterinary profession. Only undergraduate students are accepted.

Contact: DVM Admissions Office at Blacksburg campus.

UNIVERSITY OF WISCONSIN

Program: Pre-College Enrollment Opportunity Program for Learning Excellence (PEOPLE)

Description: This program began in the summer of 1999 as a partnership between the Milwaukee Public Schools and the UW-Madison with a group of students who had just completed the ninth grade. Partner schools now also include Madison high schools as well as a number of Northern Wisconsin high schools. The program is designed with a precollege track and a bridge program to undergraduate work and continues through a student's undergraduate career at University of Wisconsin-Madison. The main purposes are to promote academic preparation, increase enrollment in postsecondary institutions, and improve retention and graduation rates of minority and disadvantaged students.

Eligibility: PEOPLE is designed for students with strong academic potential who are U.S. citizens or permanent residents who are also African American, American Indian, Asian American (with an emphasis on Southeast Asian American), Chicano/a, Puerto Rican, Latino/a, or low-income students. Priority for admission will be given to students eligible for the free and reduced hot lunch program.

Program dates: June–July summer residential programs and year-round nonresidential programs.

Contact: PEOPLE Program, 1305 Linden Drive, University of Wisconsin- Madison, Madison, WI 53706.

FINANCIAL AID INFORMATION

Financing your veterinary medical education requires careful planning, good money management skills, and a willingness to make short-term sacrifices to achieve long-range goals.

Many of you will apply for and receive some type of financial assistance during your undergraduate education. This will help you become somewhat familiar with the process, and to know that the rules and regulations governing programs can and do change periodically.

As a professional student, you will be entering a partnership with the financial aid office, which will require you to complete the appropriate financial aid forms accurately, meet required deadlines, and submit any additional information that may be requested. In return, the financial aid office will determine your aid eligibility and make awards based on the available programs. Your financial aid eligibility takes into account the cost of your education minus any other available resources. Amounts of assistance and the school policies for awarding assistance vary from one veterinary medical school to another and from year to year.

Any questions or concerns that you may have about this topic need to be directed to each of the appropriate financial aid offices to ensure that you receive accurate information and guidance.

> Don't live the lifestyle of a DVM until you have completed your education. Get in the habit of being thrifty.

FINANCING YOUR VETERINARY MEDICAL EDUCATION

Your education is one of the biggest investments you will make in your lifetime, and one of your most important goals should be to maximize the return on all of your investments. To reach this goal, you must take an active role in managing your financial resources. You need to understand and implement good financial practices. To get you started, here are some good financial habits you should adopt:

- Do not use credit cards to extend your lifestyle. Deciding not to use credit cards except in emergencies is one of the most important decisions you can make, and one that will reduce your stress while you are pursuing your education.
- Budget your money just as carefully as you budget your time. Contact a financial aid administrator to help you set up a budget that will be easy to follow.
- Distinguish between wants and needs. Before you make any purchase, you should ask yourself, "Do I need this, or do I want it?"
- Be a well-informed borrower. If you have not previously taken an active role in understanding the differences between various student loan programs, now is the time to do it. You need to know these differences in order to avoid high-interest loans and to borrow wisely.
- Borrow the minimum amount necessary in order to maximize the return on your educational investment.
- Be thrifty. Live as cheaply as you can. Remember, you are a student. You'll enjoy a more comfortable lifestyle once you are a DVM.
- Pay any interest that accrues on student loans if you can afford to do so, rather than let the interest accrue and capitalize. Any amount you pay while you're a student will save you money once you enter repayment.

What is the most important piece of advice for making the most of your educational investment? Don't live the lifestyle of a DVM until you have completed your education. Get in the habit of being thrifty. If you live like a DVM while you are in school, you may have to live like a student when you are a DVM.

FEDERAL LOAN PROGRAMS

Please note that subsidized loans are not available beginning fall 2012.

	William D. Ford Unsubsidized Stafford Loan	Perkins Loan	Health Professions Student Loan	Loan for Disadvantaged Students	Grad Plus Loans for Graduate/ Professional Students
Lender	Federal Loan Program	Federal Loan Program	Federal Loan Program	Federal Loan Program	Federal Loan Program
Financial Need	No	Yes	Yes	Yes	No
Citizenship Requirement	U.S. Citizen, U.S. National, or U.S. Permanent Resident	U.S. Citizen, U.S. National, or U.S. Permanent Resident	U.S. Citizen, U.S. National, or U.S. Permanent Resident	U.S. Citizen, U.S. National, or U.S. Permanent Resident	U.S. Citizen, U.S. National, or U.S. Permanent Resident
Borrowing Limits	Cost of attendance minus other aid; $189,125 aggregate undergraduate and graduate	$6,000/year; $40,000 aggregate undergraduate and graduate	Cost of attendance at participating school	Federal Loan Programs	Cost of attendance minus other aid
Interest Rate	Fixed; capped at 6.8%	5%	5%	5%	7%
Interest Accrues While Enrolled in School	Yes	No	No	No	Yes
Deferments	Yes	Yes	Yes	Yes	Yes
Grace Period	Yes	Yes	Yes	Yes	No

A GUIDE TO PREPARING FOR VETERINARY SCHOOL

Maybe you already know that you have a strong interest in veterinary medicine, but you don't know where to start. It's never too early to begin preparing. Below are a few guidelines to help you plan your coursework and get in touch with mentors and other professionals who can help you along the way.

HIGH SCHOOL STUDENTS

- Take science and math classes, including chemistry, biology, and algebra. If available, take Advanced Placement (AP) coursework. Note, AP courses may not always satisfy vet college prerequisite coursework, but they will give you the highest level of preparation. Consult with the vet colleges to understand if AP credit in high school will satisfy a prerequisite course requirement.
- Talk to people in the field. Call local veterinarians or contact a veterinary society in your city or town to find people who can help answer your questions.
- Gain animal experiences. These will give you a good understanding of working with animals and excellent references when you seek a volunteer experience or internship with a veterinarian. Examples include volunteering at a humane society, cleaning stables and grooming horses, doing an internship at a zoo, volunteering at a nature or wildlife center, or getting involved with 4-H, just to name a few.
- Visit veterinary college websites and perhaps make a visit during one of their admissions presentations or during an open house. The more you know early on, the better prepared you will be.
- Get on the veterinary college's mailing lists for admissions updates and invitations to programs.

COLLEGE YEAR 1

Fall semester
- Obtain a copy of the *AAVMC Veterinary Medical School Admission Requirements* (*VMSAR*) to review the veterinary schools' requirements with your advisor.
- Meet with an advisor and plan coursework. Take the list of prerequisite courses on the AAVMC website or in *VMSAR* for planning purposes. Not all vet colleges require the exact same courses, but most will want courses in the areas of biology, chemistry, and physics. That's a good place to start until you narrow down your list of vet colleges to apply to.
- Start working on the prerequisite coursework. Most vet colleges require quite a few biology and chemistry courses. Starting out right away in these introductory courses will allow you to move forward quickly.

Spring semester
- Think about summer volunteer or employment opportunities in veterinary medicine, such as shadowing a veterinarian or volunteering in an animal shelter.
- Continue working on the introductory courses and register for the fall semester.
- Research preveterinary enrichment programs at ExploreHealthCareers.org. Preveterinary enrichment programs can help you decide if a career in veterinary medicine is a good fit and help prepare you for the application process.

Summer
- Complete an internship or volunteer program.
- Attend summer school, if necessary. Note, many vet colleges prefer the prerequisite coursework be taken in a full-time load during the academic year. If possible, take general education or major courses during the summer.

COLLEGE YEAR 2

Fall semester
- Meet with your advisor to discuss your progress.
- Attend preveterinary activities.
- Join your school's preveterinary society, if one is available.
- Continue working on prerequisite coursework.
- Explore community service opportunities through your school (they don't necessarily need to be animal-related). If possible, continue activities throughout undergraduate career.

Spring semester
- Look into paid or volunteer veterinary-related research opportunities.
- Complete second semester coursework and register for the fall.

Summer
- Complete a summer research or volunteer veterinary-related program.
- Attend summer school, if necessary.
- Prepare for the Graduate Record Examination (GRE).

- Visit veterinary colleges. Meet with someone from the admissions office or attend an admissions presentation and take a tour.

COLLEGE YEAR 3

Fall semester

- Meet with your preveterinary advisor.
- Discuss veterinary schools.
- Register for spring semester.
- Visit the AAVMC's website (www.aavmc.org) to learn about applying to veterinary schools.
- Place your order for the *AAVMC Veterinary Medical School Admission Requirements*.
- Research schools.

Spring semester

- Identify individuals (veterinarian, faculty member or advisor, supervisor of animal experiences, research faculty) to write letters of recommendation.
- Take the GRE during late spring or early summer.
- Prepare to submit your vet school applications.
- Register for the fall semester.
- Schedule a volunteer or paid veterinary medicine-related activity.

Summer

- Take the GRE if you have not done so already.
- Budget time and finances appropriately to attend interviews.
- Participate in a volunteer or paid opportunity.
- Attend summer school, if necessary.
- Work on and submit your applications. Most vet colleges have a supplemental application, so be very careful to meet **all deadlines** for the VMCAS application, supplemental application, and getting in supporting documentation and letters.

COLLEGE YEAR 4

Fall semester

- Meet with your advisor.
- Attend interviews with schools.
- Notification of acceptances begins December 1.

Spring semester

- Apply for federal financial aid.
- April 15 deadline to let the vet colleges where you have been admitted know your decision.

Summer

- Attend school's orientation.
- Prepare to relocate, if necessary.

VETERINARY MEDICAL COLLEGE APPLICATION SERVICE (VMCAS)

The Veterinary Medical College Application Service is a centralized application service sponsored by the Association of American Veterinary Medical Colleges. Applicants use VMCAS to apply to most of the AVMA-accredited colleges in the United States and abroad.

VMCAS collects, processes, and ships application materials to veterinary colleges designated by the applicant, and responds to applicant inquiries about the application process. This service is the data collection, processing, and distribution component of the admission process for colleges participating in VMCAS. VMCAS, however, does not take part in the admissions selection process.

Twenty-nine (29) of the thirty (30) U.S. veterinary institutions participate in VMCAS, along with two (2) Canadian, two (2) Scottish, one (1) English, one (1) Irish, two (2) Australian, and one (1) New Zealand veterinary institutions. Application material deadlines, prerequisite courses, and other aspects of the admissions process differ from school to school. Applicants are responsible for being informed of all instructions provided by VMCAS and the associated member colleges. Questions about using VMCAS should be directed to the VMCAS Student and Advisor Hotline.

APPLICATION CYCLE TIMELINE

VMCAS launch: May 11, 2018
VMCAS Application Deadline: September 17, 2018, 12 Midnight Eastern Time
AAVMC Acceptance Deadline: April 16, 2019
Please be sure to verify individual school deadlines

KEY ONLINE RESOURCES

General Information Chart

A one-stop comparison of school info such as location, tuition, seat availability, etc.
http://aavmc.org/data/files/vmcas/geninfochart.pdf

Prerequisite Comparison Chart

A course requirement comparison chart of all AAVMC member schools.
http://aavmc.org/data/files/vmcas/prereqchart.pdf

Fee Structure

VMCAS fees broken down by number of designations.
http://aavmc.org/Applicant-Responsibilities/Fees.aspx

Evaluation Requirements

Individual recommendation requirements by school.
www.aavmc.org/Applicant-Responsibilities/Evaluations.aspx

VMCAS

655 K Street, NW Suite 725
Washington, DC 20001
Telephone: (617) 612-2884
Fax: (617) 612-2051
vmcasinfo@vmcas.org
www.aavmc.org

VETERINARY MEDICAL SCHOOLS
IN THE **UNITED STATES**
COE Accredited

AUBURN UNIVERSITY

Email Address: admissions@vetmed.auburn.edu
Website: www.vetmed.auburn.edu

AUBURN UNIVERSITY

COLLEGE OF VETERINARY MEDICINE

SCHOOL DESCRIPTION

The College of Veterinary Medicine at Auburn University is located in south central Alabama off Interstate 85 between Montgomery and Atlanta. The college is known for its friendly small-campus atmosphere.

Veterinary medicine began as a department at Auburn in 1892 and became a college in 1907. Today it is situated on 330 acres one mile from the main Auburn campus that serves more than 28,000 students. In addition, the college has a 700-acre research farm five miles from its campus. The college is fully accredited by the American Veterinary Medical Association.

> Students have the opportunity to work with more than 100 nationally and internationally recognized faculty.

APPLICATION INFORMATION

For specific application information (availability, deadlines, fees, and VMCAS participation), please refer to the contact information listed above.

Residency implications: 41 Alabama residents, 38 Kentucky residents, and 41 non-contract non-resident students.

Required undergraduate GPA: Alabama and Kentucky residents must have a minimum grade point average of 2.50 on a 4.00 scale. Applicants not classified as Alabama or Kentucky residents must have a minimum grade point average of 3.00 on a 4.00 scale. A grade of C-minus or better must be earned for any required course. The mean grade point average of the most recent entering class was 3.60.

AP credit policy: must appear on official college transcripts and be equivalent to the appropriate college-level coursework.

Course completion deadline: prerequisite courses must be completed by June 15 prior to matriculation.

Standardized examinations: Graduate Record Examination (GRE®), general test, is required. The exam must have been taken within the previous 5 calendar years, and must be received no later than September 15 of the year of application, therefore you should test no later than September 1.

GRE Code: 1005

ADDITIONAL REQUIREMENTS AND CONSIDERATIONS

A minimum of 500 hours of veterinary experience in addition to other animal experience

Recommendations (3 required)
    Academic advisor or faculty member
    Employer
    Veterinarian

Extracurricular and community service activities

Narrative statement of purpose

SUMMARY OF ADMISSION PROCEDURES

VMCAS application deadline: Monday, September 17, 2018 at 12 Midnight Eastern Time

Date interviews are held: Non-contract, non-resident February; Alabama and Kentucky residents March

Date acceptances mailed: Within 12 days following interviews

PREREQUISITES FOR ADMISSION

Course Requirements	Number of Semester Hours
Written composition#	6
* Literature#	3
Fine Arts#	3
Humanities/fine arts elective#	6
* History#	3
Social/behavioral science electives#	9
Mathematics—precalculus with trigonometry#	3
Biology I with lab	4
Biology II with lab	4
***Cell Biology	3
Fundamentals of chemistry with lab	8
Organic chemistry 1 with lab; Organic chemistry 2	6
Physics I	4
Biochemistry	3
Science electives**	6
Animal Nutrition##	3

* Students must complete a 6-semester-hour sequence either in literature or in history.

** Science electives must be two of the following: genetics, microbiology, physics II, comparative anatomy, histology, reproductive physiology, mammalian or animal physiology, parasitology, embryology, or immunology.

*** The cell biology course, beyond an introductory biology course, should focus on the molecular biology of cells, membranes, cytoplasm, and organelles as well as energy, transport, motility, cell division, signaling, transcription, and translation. Microbiology, genetics, physiology, or other courses may not be used to fulfill the cell biology requirement.

These requirements will be waived if the student has a bachelor's degree.

Will accept web based or correspondence course. Animal nutrition must focus on large animal, small animal, monogastric, and ruminant species.

School begins: August

Deposit (to hold place in class): none required

Deferments: not considered

Transfer Students: Auburn does not take transfer students

International Students: not considered for admission

Evaluation criteria: Auburn University has a three-part admission procedure: an objective evaluation of academic credentials; a subjective review of personal credentials and experience under veterinary supervision; and a personal interview.

2017–2018 ADMISSIONS SUMMARY

Number of Applicants
Resident: 90
Contract*: 116
Non-resident: 741
Total: 943

Number of New Entrants
Resident: 41
Contract*: 38
Non-resident: 41
Total: 120

ESTIMATED TUITION

Tuition and fees
Resident: $20,060
Non-resident: $46,748
Contract*: $20,060

* For further information, see the listing of contracting states and provinces (see pg. 12).

** Please be aware that the estimated cost of attendance is higher for the third academic year when a summer semester is required because of the continuous year of clinical training.

ENTRANCE REQUIREMENTS

Admitted students fall into three categories: residents of Alabama, residents of Kentucky admitted by contract through the Southern Regional Education Board (SREB), or at-large residents (non-Alabama and non-contract students).

Kentucky students must verify their residency status with their Kentucky pre-vet advisor before September 15. They may contact the Kentucky Council on Postsecondary Education for additional information.

Resident/contract applicants must be a documented resident of Alabama or Kentucky.

ADDITIONAL INFORMATION

Application Deadline: 9/17/2018

UNIVERSITY OF CALIFORNIA

Email Address: admissions@vetmed.ucdavis.edu
Website: www.vetmed.ucdavis.edu

SCHOOL DESCRIPTION

The University of California, Davis (UC Davis) campus is one of 10 campuses of the University of California system. It is the largest campus, with 5,300 acres. The Davis campus is located in Yolo County in the Central Valley of Northern California. Davis is situated 11 miles west of Sacramento, 385 miles north of Los Angeles, and 72 miles northeast of San Francisco. Davis is surrounded by open space, including some of the most productive agricultural land in the state. The terrain is flat and the City of Davis is a friendly college town that cares about sustainability and welcoming newcomers. Ranked as one of the best towns to live in in the nation, Davis is also considered the most bike-friendly city in the nation. The Central Valley climate can be described as Mediterranean. The mild temperate climate means enjoyment of outdoors all year long. During the hot, dry, sunny summers, temperatures on some days can exceed 100 degrees F; however, more often summer temperatures are in the low 90s. Spring and fall has some of the most pleasant weather in the state. Winters in Davis are usually mild. UC Davis is an outstanding research and training institution with over 35,000 undergraduate, graduate and professional students. The Davis campus has four undergraduate colleges, graduate studies in all schools and colleges, and six professional programs carried out in the schools of Education, Law, Management, Medicine, Nursing, and Veterinary Medicine.

> UC Davis is an outstanding research and training institution with over 35,000 students.

Since 1948 the School of Veterinary Medicine serves the people of California by providing educational, research, clinical service, and public service programs of the highest quality to advance the health and care of animals, the public, and the environment. School of Veterinary Medicine faculty members have earned a reputation for their broad expertise and shared commitment to solving some of society's most persistent health problems. The school's impact is evident in the accomplishments of clinicians who have developed novel treatments and basic scientists who continue to make major discoveries in animal, human and environmental health. We address the health of all animals, including livestock, poultry, companion animals, captive and free-ranging wildlife, exotic animals, birds, aquatic mammals and fish, and animals used in biological and medical research. Our expertise also encompasses related human health concerns.

To carry out this mission, we focus on students in our professional Doctor of Veterinary Medicine program, Master of Preventive Veterinary Medicine program, graduate clinical residency program and graduate academic MS and PhD programs. The school is fully committed to recruiting students with diverse backgrounds.

The School of Veterinary Medicine is home of the William R. Pritchard Veterinary Medical Teaching Hospital, Veterinary Medicine Teaching and Research Center, California Animal Health and Food Safety Laboratory, UC Veterinary Medical Center-San Diego and Centers of Excellence-fostering research, teaching and service focused on species interests and multidisciplinary themes. There are many other centers and innovative programs at UC Davis. Our statewide mission includes 28 research and clinical programs including continuing education; extension; and community outreach.

PREREQUISITES FOR ADMISSION

Course Description	Number of Hours/Credits	Necessity
General chemistry (with laboratory)	Two semesters (3 quarters) w/lab	Required
Organic chemistry (with laboratory)	Two semesters (2-3 quarters) w/lab	Required
Physics	Two semesters (2-3 quarters)	Required
General biology (with laboratory)	Two semesters (3 quarters) w/lab	Required
*Systemic physiology	One semester/quarter	Required
*Biochemistry (bioenergetics and metabolism)	One semester/quarter	Required
*Genetics (genes and gene expression)	One semester/quarter	Required
Statistics	One semester/quarter	Required

*courses must be taken at the upper division level at a four-year university.

APPLICATION INFORMATION

For specific application information (availability, deadlines, fees, and VMCAS participation), please refer to our website at www.vetmed.ucdavis.edu.

Residency implications: A nonspecified number of resident and nonresident applicants are accepted. International applicants are also considered for admission. (Please note: Beginning with the 2018-2019 application cycle, WICHE applicants will be considered nonresidents.)

SUMMARY OF ADMISSION PROCEDURES

VMCAS application deadline: Monday, September 17, 2018 at 9 PM Pacific Time

Supplemental information is required. School will notify the applicant to set-up portal and complete supplemental information after application has been verified by VMCAS.

Date interviews are held: TBD (December or January)

Date admission notifications available in portal: TBD (January or February)

School begins: August

Deposit (to hold place in class): not required

Deferments: reviewed on a case-by-case basis for unexpected medical reasons or situations beyond control of applicant

EVALUATION CRITERIA

Cumulative Science GPA

Last (most recent) 45 semester/67.5 quarter units GPA

GRE Quantitative scores

VMCAS Electronic Letters of Recommendation (eLOR)

MMI Interview

ENTRANCE REQUIREMENTS

Required undergraduate GPA: a minimum grade point average of 2.50 on a 4.00 scale is required for all science courses completed and 2.50 on all courses cumulatively at time of application. Applicants admitted in fall 2017 had a mean cumulative GPA of 3.70 and a mean science GPA of 3.71.

AP credit policy: Credit must appear on official college transcript with course name and units awarded and must be equivalent to the prerequisite course being satisfied.

Is a Bachelor's Degree Required? yes

Is this an International School? no

ESTIMATED TUITION

Estimated Tuition Resident: $36,011

Estimated Tuition Contract: n/a

Estimated Tuition Non-Resident: $48,256

AVAILABLE SEATS - 150

Resident: varied

Contract: n/a

Non-Resident: varied

TEST REQUIREMENTS

Standardized examinations: Graduate Record Examination, general test is required. The acceptable GRE test dates for applicants entering 2019 are August 31, 2013

- August 31, 2018. Scores must be sent directly to VMCAS code 4804 by September 17, 2018.

VMCAS Participation: full

Accepts International Students? yes

ADDITIONAL INFORMATION

Dual-Degree Programs

Combined DVM/PhD graduate degree programs are available.

Visit our Veterinary Scientist Training Program information at www.vetmed.ucdavis.edu/vstp/index.cfm.

Application Deadline: 9/17/2018

COLORADO STATE UNIVERSITY

Email Address: dvmadmissions@colostate.edu
Website: csu-cvmbs.colostate.edu/dvm-program
/Pages/DVM-Program-Entrance-Requirements.aspx

DOCTOR OF VETERINARY MEDICINE PROGRAM

SCHOOL DESCRIPTION

Colorado State University is located in Fort Collins, a city of about 150,000 in the eastern foothills of the Rocky Mountains about 65 miles north of Denver. Fort Collins has a pleasant climate and offers many cultural and recreational activities. Many of the state's ski areas lie within a short driving distance, making some of the best skiing in the world accessible. The nearby river canyons and mountain parks are beautiful scenic attractions and provide opportunities for hiking, fishing, photography, camping, and biking.

> Colorado State University is located in Fort Collins, a city of about 150,000 in the eastern foothills of the Rockies.

The College of Veterinary Medicine and Biomedical Sciences is nationally renowned for its programs in oncology, equine surgery and reproduction, and pain management. Our college is composed of eight major buildings that house the departments of biomedical sciences, environmental and radiological health sciences, and microbiology, immunology, and pathology.

The James L. Voss Veterinary Teaching Hospital, one of the world's largest and best equipped, houses the clinical sciences department. This department boasts a variety of unique units, including the internationally acclaimed Robert H. and Mary G. Flint Animal Cancer Center, Integrated Livestock Management Program, Gail Holmes Equine Orthopaedic Research Center, and C. Wayne McIlwraith Translational Medicine Institute. The hospital attracts a large caseload and offers students a wide variety of clinical experiences.

The uniquely designed Diagnostic Medicine Center houses the college's Veterinary Diagnostic Laboratory (VDL), the University's Extension Veterinarian, the Clinical Pathology Laboratory and the Animal Population Health Institute.

The VDL provides disease testing services to veterinarians, state/federal agencies, livestock owners and pet owners. The Clinical Pathology Laboratory provides services such as blood, fluid and urine analysis and cytology to identify diseases and illnesses in animals brought to the VTH or to veterinarians in the region. The Animal Population Health Institute encourages collaboration and information and expertise exchange in veterinary epidemiology among scientists at CSU, collaborating institutions and government agencies throughout the world.

Internationally known for its innovative curriculum, our veterinary program provides students with a four-year course of study in veterinary medicine leading to the Doctor of Veterinary Medicine degree. The first two years are conducted on the main campus and include comprehensive coverage of veterinary and biomedical sciences along with integrated hands-on and clinical experiences. During the second two years, students participate in animal care at the Veterinary Teaching Hospital through a series of specialty rotations. Students participate as team members in evaluating patients, meeting with clients, developing treatment plans, and providing hands-on care, all under the supervision of faculty clinicians.

PREREQUISITES FOR ADMISSION

Course Description	Number of Semester Credits	Necessity
Biochemistry (that requires Org Chem)	3	Required
Genetics (that requires biology)	3	Required
Physics (with a laboratory)	4	Required
Statistics	3	Required
Lab associated with a biology course	1	Required
Lab associated with a chemistry course	1	Required
English Composition (or completion of four-year degree)	3	Required
Social sciences and humanities	12	Required
Electives	30	Required
Upper level biomedical sciences		Recommended

APPLICATION INFORMATION

Application requirements: For your application to be reviewed by the Veterinary Admissions Committee, we must receive the following items before the deadline:

- VMCAS Application, three VMCAS eLORs, and Fee
- Colorado Supplemental Application (CSA) and Fee
- GRE Verbal, Quantitative, and Analytical (self-reported unofficial scores in the CSA)

SUMMARY OF ADMISSION PROCEDURES

Colorado Supplemental Application deadline: Monday, September 17, 2018 at 10 PM (MT). Fee: $80

VMCAS application deadline: Monday, September 17, 2018 at 12 Midnight (ET)

School begins: late August

Deposit: (to hold place in class) none required

Deferments: case-by-case basis for extenuating circumstances

EVALUATION CRITERIA

- Quality of academic program (course load, challenging curriculum, honors)
- GRE scores
- Veterinary/Animal/Research/Work Employment experience

- Extracurricular/Community/Leadership activities and achievements
- Personal Essay
- Contribution to diversity, unique attributes, extenuating circumstances
- Letters of Reference, three VMCAS eLORs - veterinarian, academic, employment - with at least one being from a veterinarian

ENTRANCE REQUIREMENTS

Required undergraduate GPA: No minimum requirement

Mean GPA: for the 2017 matriculated class was 3.70 on a 4.00 scale

AP credits: must appear on official transcript

Course completion deadline: final grades/transcripts, including all required courses, must be received at CSU by July 15 prior to matriculation

Is a Bachelor's Degree Required? no

Is this an International School? no

ESTIMATED TUITION

Estimated Tuition Resident: $34,000

Estimated Tuition Contract: $34,000

Estimated Tuition Non-Resident: $59,000

AVAILABLE SEATS

Resident: 70

Non-resident: 30-35

Contract: 30-35

UAF/CSU: 10

TEST REQUIREMENTS

The GRE General Test (Verbal, Quantitative, Analytical) is required. The average GRE scores for the 2017 matriculated class are in the mid-150's for Verbal and Quantitative; and in the range of 4.0-4.5 for Analytical.

Test scores must be dated on or after August 1, 2013. It is the applicant's responsibility to schedule the test on or before August 13, 2018, so they can self-report unofficial scores on the Colorado Supplemental Application before the September 17, 2018, at 10:00 PM (MT) deadline. NOTE: The self-reported unofficial scores—Verbal, Quantitative, and Analytical—must be entered into the Colorado Supplemental Application in order to submit the application.

Sending official scores: Applicants should submit a request to their testing center, before September 15, to have official scores sent to CSU (code 4075; dept 0617). Official scores should be received at CSU by October 31. Official scores will be used to verify all applicant self-reported scores before offers are made.

VMCAS Participation: full

Accepts International Students? yes

ADDITIONAL INFORMATION

The veterinary program at CSU offers the following programs:

UAF (Alaska)/CSU: http://csu-cvmbs.colostate.edu/dvm-program/Pages/uaf-csu-collaborative-veterinary-program.aspx

MBA/DVM: http://csu-cvmbs.colostate.edu/dvm-program/Pages/DVM-MBA.aspx

MPH/DVM: http://csu-cvmbs.colostate.edu/dvm-program/Pages/DVM-MPH.aspx

MSA/DVM: http://csu-cvmbs.colostate.edu/dvm-program/Pages/dvm-msansci.aspx

MST/DVM: http://csu-cvmbs.colostate.edu/dvm-program/Pages/DVM-MST.aspx

PhD/DVM: http://csu-cvmbs.colostate.edu/dvm-program/Pages/DVM-PhD.aspx

FAVCIP (Food Animal): http://csu-cvmbs.colostate.edu/dvm-program/Pages/DVM-Special-Programs.aspx

Application Deadline: 9/17/2018

VETERINARIAN PROFILE: JIMMY JOHNSON

YEAR OF GRADUATION
2012

PLACE OF EMPLOYMENT
Columbus Zoo and Aquarium

What is your favorite aspect of being a veterinarian?
My favorite aspect of being a veterinarian is the versatility of our profession, combining general medical care, problem-solving, and scientific inquiry with a variety of animal species, especially in my specialty of zoological medicine. Veterinarians are professionals who work at the interface of animal and human health, as well as ecosystem health and conservation, making our work meaningful and rewarding in the clinic, the lab, society, or in nature.

What type of veterinary medicine do you practice?
I am a specialist in zoological medicine, board-certified by the American College of Zoological Medicine. I practice as a staff veterinarian at the Columbus Zoo and Aquarium, and I serve as an adjunct assistant professor in the Department of Veterinary Preventative Medicine at the Ohio State University College of Veterinary Medicine.

Where did you attend veterinary school?
The Ohio State University.

How long have you been practicing as a veterinarian?
Five-and-half years.

What advice do you have for those considering a career in veterinary medicine?
Veterinary medicine offers many diverse opportunities. Students interested in pursuing a career veterinary medicine should take the time to explore these opportunities and understand the breadth of this field, and wildlife and conservation medicine, among many other disciplines. Veterinarians are versatile health professionals, so a demonstrated effort to explore the many facets of this profession, along with striving for high academic standards and participating in diverse activities, can develop a student into a competitive applicant for veterinary school. Students should know that investing in their education and exploring their interests can genuinely help them achieve their dreams. Veterinary training requires a substantial obligation of time and effort, but it is an exciting adventure where lasting friendships can be made and valuable professional and personal skills can be attained, ultimately resulting in a fulfilling and meaningful career as a veterinarian.

What challenges have you faced while practicing veterinary medicine?
Veterinary medicine requires good mental aptitude to be able to manage a variety of challenges and questions daily regarding such things as patient care, scientific investigation, business management, and communication with colleagues and clients. In addition, physical demands can vary depending on the field of veterinary medicine, but in my practice, it takes the strength of a team to move an anesthetized rhinoceros or very fine motor skills to perform microsurgery on a hamster. Veterinarian salaries are not as high as our human physician counterparts, especially compared to the student loan debt that can be financially taxing. However, I am still able to make a living doing a job that I really enjoy.

CORNELL UNIVERSITY

Email Address: vet_admissions@cornell.edu
Website: www.vet.cornell.edu/admissions

SCHOOL DESCRIPTION

Cornell is located in Ithaca, a college town of about 30,000 in the Finger Lakes region of upstate New York, a beautiful area of rolling hills, deep valleys, scenic gorges, and clear lakes. The university's 740-acre campus is bounded on two sides by gorges and waterfalls. Open countryside, state parks, and year-round opportunities for outdoor recreation, including excellent sailing, swimming, skiing, hiking, and other activities, are only minutes away.

Ithaca is one hour by air and a four-hour drive from New York City, and other major metropolitan areas are easily accessible. Direct commercial flights connect Ithaca with New York, Philadelphia, and Detroit airport hubs.

The tradition of academic excellence, the cultural vigor of a distinguished university, and the magnificent setting create a stimulating environment for graduate study. The curriculum differs from other programs in that it is interdisciplinary, small group learning early in the program and focuses on the student as the primary force in learning.

> The curriculum is interdisciplinary and focuses on the student as the primary force in learning.

APPLICATION INFORMATION

For specific information about the application process visit our web site at: http://www.vet.cornell.edu/admissions

You may also subscribe to our free electronic Pre-Vet Newsletter at: http://www.vet.cornell.edu/admissions/PreVetNewsletters.cfm for application updates and current information about the College of Veterinary Medicine.

Residency implications: approximately 66 seats for New York State residents and 54 seats for non-NY residents

SUMMARY OF ADMISSION PROCEDURES

VMCAS application deadline: Monday, September 17, 2018 at 12 Midnight Eastern Time

Date acceptances emailed: January

Information sessions at the college for admitted students and alternates: February

School begins: mid/late August

Deposit (to hold place in class): $500.00 (by April 15, unless the 15th falls on a weekend, then the deposit deadline will be the following Monday)

Deferments: considered on an individual basis, and ordinarily granted for illness or other situations beyond the control of the applicant.

EVALUATION CRITERIA

The following admissions formula allows the applicant to see how their application will be reviewed:

25% Overall GPA

25% GRE (verbal & quantitative) or MCAT Scores

20% Animal/Veterinary/Biomedical Research Experiences

PREREQUISITES FOR ADMISSION

Course Description	Number of Semester Credits	Necessity
English composition/writing-intensive courses (full year)	6	Required
Biology or zoology, full year with laboratory	6	Required
Physics, full year with laboratory	6	Required
Inorganic (or general) chemistry, full year with laboratory	6	Required
Organic chemistry, one semester	3	Required
Biochemistry, half year required; full year preferred	4	Required
Advanced Life Science course	3	Required
Non-prerequisite elective credits needed	26	Required

• at least one letter of evaluation from a veterinarian is required

5% Quality of Academic Program

• with academic letter of evaluation

10% Non-Cognitive Skills

10% All Other Achievements

5% Personal Statement

ENTRANCE REQUIREMENTS

Required undergraduate GPA: No specific GPA requirement, but the grade range of those admitted tends to be 3.00-4.00.

AP credit policy: accepted for physics and general or inorganic chemistry with a score of 4 or higher.

Course completion deadline: all but 12 semester credits (or 18 quarter credits) of the prerequisite coursework should be completed at the time of application, with at least one semester of any two-semester series underway. Any outstanding prerequisites must be completed by the end of the spring term prior to matriculation.

Is a Bachelor's Degree Required? no

Is this an International School? no

ESTIMATED TUITION

Estimated Tuition Resident: $34,750

Estimated Tuition Contract: n/a

Estimated Tuition Non-Resident: $50,980

AVAILABLE SEATS

Resident: tentative 66

Contract: 0

Non-Resident: tentative 54

TEST REQUIREMENTS

Standardized examinations: Graduate Record Examination (GRE), general test (verbal and quantitative), or the Medical College Admission Test (MCAT) is required. Official test scores must be received directly from ETS or AAVMC by the September deadline. Test scores older than five years will not be accepted. TOEFL scores for international applicants whose first language is not English (and whose education was taught in a language other than English) should be received by this deadline as well.

VMCAS Participation: full

Accepts International Students? yes

ADDITIONAL INFORMATION

Combined Degree Programs

Combined DVM/PhD Program: By integrating Cornell's veterinary and graduate curricula in the DVM/ PhD Program, we prepare students to become leaders in science, medicine, and society, able to excel in basic research, cutting-edge medicine, and teaching. Students receive substantial financial funding incentives to complete both degrees.

DVM/MPH (Masters in Public Health): A partnership between the College of Veterinary Medicine and the University Of Minnesota School Of Public Health allows students the opportunity to earn a Master of Public Health (MPH) degree while completing their DVM training.

For more information on both combined degree programs visit: http://www.vet.cornell.edu/admissions/OADualDegree.cfm

Other Admissions Programs

Sophomore Early Acceptance Program: The Early Acceptance Program gives exceptionally well qualified applicants the opportunity to obtain admission to veterinary school after the completion of the sophomore year and start the veterinary curriculum after completion of the junior year. With admission to the Cornell University College of Veterinary Medicine secured, the successful applicant may use the time between acceptance and matriculation to pursue experience in areas of personal interest. More information can be found at: https://www2 .vet.cornell.edu/education/doctorveterinary-medicine /admissions/early-acceptance

Cornell Accelerated BS/DVM Program: Joint program between the College of Agriculture and Life Sciences and the College of Veterinary Medicine at Cornell University. A seven-year BS/DVM program for those looking for an accelerated path to a veterinary degree. More information can be found at https://www2.vet.cornell .edu/education/doctor-veterinary-medicine/admissions /early-admission-programs/cornell-accelerated-bsdvm -program

Transfer Student Admissions: Cornell will consider applications for advanced standing in the DVM program on an individual basis, if an opening exists in the second-year class. More information can be found at: http://www.vet.cornell.edu/admissions/transfer_students.cfm

Summer Research Opportunities

The Leadership Program for Veterinary Scholars: A unique summer learning experience for veterinary students who seek to broadly influence the veterinary profession through a career in research. The program in an intensive research-oriented learning experience that combines faculty-guided research with career counseling, student-directed learning, and a variety of professional enrichment activities.

Additional Summer Research Opportunities: Additional summer research opportunities for veterinary students include the Veterinary Investigator Program, Veterinary Training in Biomedical Research, Aquavet, Summer Dairy Institute, the Food Animal Medicine Externship, and the Havemeyer Foundation Equine Research Fellowships.

For more information about all of these summer research opportunities visit: http://www.vet.cornell.edu/BBS/Scientists /SummerResearch.cfm

Other

Masters in Public Health at Cornell University: Beginning fall 2017 a campus-wide MPH program. Founded on the One Health paradigm. For more information: https:// www2.vet.cornell.edu/education/graduate-studies /master-public-health-mph.

Master of Professional Studies-Veterinary Parasitology. This MPS program is designed for individuals who seek to enhance their careers with specialized professional training in Veterinary Parasitology. For more information: https://www2.vet.cornell.edu/education/graduate -studies/master-professional-studies-parasitology

Application Deadline: VMCAS 9/17/2018

UNIVERSITY OF FLORIDA

Email Address: studentservices@vetmed.ufl.edu
Website: www.vetmed.ufl.edu

UF | UNIVERSITY *of* FLORIDA

SCHOOL DESCRIPTION

The University of Florida is located in Gainesville, a college town of approximately 125,000 in north central Florida, midway between the Gulf of Mexico and the Atlantic Ocean. Changes in season are marked, but winters are mild and permit year-round participation in outdoor activities.

The university accommodates about 50,000+ students with programs in almost all disciplines. The College of Veterinary Medicine is a component of the Institute of Food and Agricultural Sciences (which also includes Agriculture and Forest Resources and Conservation). It is also one of 6 colleges affiliated with the Health Science Center (the other 5 are Dentistry, Public Health and Health Professions, Medicine, Nursing, and Pharmacy).

> The veterinary curriculum is a 9-semester program consisting of core curriculum and elective experiences.

The veterinary curriculum is a 9-semester program consisting of core curriculum and elective experiences. The core provides the body of knowledge and skills common to all veterinarians. The first four semesters concentrate primarily on basic medical sciences. In the first four semesters, students are also introduced to physical diagnosis, radiology, and clinical problems. They also spend time preparing for the clinical experience in a clinical techniques simulation laboratory and in the hospital by participating in supervised patient care. The core also includes experience in each of the specialized clinical areas and primary care. Elective areas of concentration permit students to investigate further the aspects of both basic and clinical sciences most relevant to their interests (e.g., small animal, food animal, equine, etc.). Students may also participate in optional Certificate Programs and/or the Joint DVM/MPH Program.

APPLICATION INFORMATION

For specific application information (availability, deadlines, fees, and VMCAS participation), please refer to the contact information listed above.

Residency implications: Florida has no contractual agreements. The college admits 94 Florida residents and 26 Non-Sponsored applicants each academic year. International applicants are included in the Non-Sponsored pool.

SUMMARY OF ADMISSION PROCEDURES

VMCAS application deadline: Monday, September 17, 2018 at 12 Midnight Eastern Time

UF Professional School Application deadline: Monday, September 17, 2018. Information on our supplemental requirements can be found at: http://education.vetmed.ufl.edu/admissions/application

Date interviews are held: January/February

Date acceptances mailed: March

School begins: mid-August

Deposit (to hold place in class): none required

Deferments: considered on an individual basis

PREREQUISITES FOR ADMISSION

Course Description	Number of Hours/Credits	Necessity
Biology (general, genetics, microbiology)	15	Required
Chemistry (inorganic, organic, biochemistry)	19	Required
Physics	8	Required
Mathematics (statistics)	3	Required
Humanities	9	Required
Social sciences	6	Required
English (2 courses in English composition)	6	Required
Electives	5	Required

EVALUATION CRITERIA

Academic Assessment

The University of Florida College of Veterinary Medicine (UFCVM) does not have a set minimum academic requirement in order to be admitted. However, Science, Last 45 and Overall GPAs in addition to GRE scores will be used in evaluating the academic ranking of applicants. Candidates are ranked in two independent applicant pools: Sponsored (Florida residents) and Non-Sponsored.

Full Application Review

Applicants selected from the academic ranking will have their entire vet school application reviewed individually by three members of the UFCVM Admissions Committee. Once again, there will be two applicant pools: Sponsored and Non-Sponsored, and the candidates will be scored and ranked on the following criteria:

Academic History and Experience: Academic load, number of withdrawals, research participation, teaching assistant positions, strength of academic references (if any), and academic flags/concerns.

Pre-Veterinary Experience and Preparation: Amount of legitimate pre-veterinary experience, amount of legitimate animal experience, strength of veterinary/animal-related references, relationship with references, and veterinary/animal experiences.

Overall Professionalism and Readiness to Matriculate: Overall professionalism of the application, strength of written communication skills, extracurricular experiences, community involvement, international experiences, awards and recognitions, non-veterinary or animal related employment experiences.

Candidate Interview

In early-to-mid February candidates selected from the full application review pool, will be invited to participate in the Interview process. Each applicant will be interviewed by a panel of two members of the Admissions Committee and one upper division Veterinary Student.

ENTRANCE REQUIREMENTS

Suggested undergraduate GPA: a minimum GPA of 3.00 on a 4.00 scale. The class of 2021 had an overall mean science prerequisite GPA of 3.59.

Course completion deadline: Applicants are expected to complete 80% of the Science and Math prerequisite courses before submitting an application.

Is a Bachelor's Degree Required? no

Is this an International School? no

ESTIMATED TUITION

Estimated Tuition Resident: $28,787

Estimated Tuition Contract: $0

Estimated Tuition Non-Resident: $45,500

AVAILABLE SEATS

Resident: 94

Contract: 0

Non-Resident: 26

TEST REQUIREMENTS

Standardized examinations: The Graduate Record Examination General Test is required. To be considered for Class of 2023 admissions cycle, the last day to sit for the GRE is August 31, 2018.

VMCAS Participation: full

Accepts International Students? on a case-by-case basis

ADDITIONAL INFORMATION

Supplemental Application Deadline: 9/17/2018

UNIVERSITY OF GEORGIA

Email Address: dvmadmit@uga.edu
Website: www.vet.uga.edu/admissions

UNIVERSITY OF
GEORGIA
College of
Veterinary Medicine

SCHOOL DESCRIPTION

The University of Georgia is located in Athens-Clarke County, with a population of over 100,000. Georgia's Classic City is a prospering community that reflects the charm of the Old South while growing in culture and industry (www. visitathensga.com). Athens is just over an hour away from the north Georgia mountains and the metropolitan area of Atlanta, and just over 5 hours away from the Atlantic coast.

> The University of Georgia has grown into an institution with 16 schools and colleges and more than 2,889 faculty.

In 1785, Georgia became the first state to grant a charter for a state-supported university. In 1801 the first students came to the newly formed frontier town of Athens. The University of Georgia has grown into an institution with 16 schools and colleges and more than 2,889 faculty members and 34,519 students.

APPLICATION INFORMATION

For specific application information (availability, deadlines, fees, and VMCAS participation), please refer to the contact information listed above.

Residency implications: Georgia retains up to 19 positions for contract students. Contracts are with Delaware (maximum 2 seats) and South Carolina (maximum 17 seats). The balance of those admitted are residents of Georgia or nonresident, non-contract applicants. International applications are accepted. Total number of students admitted each year: 114.

SUMMARY OF ADMISSION PROCEDURES

VMCAS application deadline: Monday, September 17, 2018 at 12 Midnight Eastern Time

Supplemental application deadline: September 17, 2018 at 1 PM Eastern Time (The deadline to request a supplemental application account will be posted on our website).

GRE score deadline: September 17, 2018 (scores must be submitted electronically from ETS) (Applicant must use code 5752).

Decision letters mailed: early–middle February

School begins: mid-August. A required 3-day orientation will precede the start of classes.

Deposit (to hold place in class): $500; $750 for nonresident, non-contract students.

Deferments: one-year deferments considered on a case-by-case basis.

EVALUATION CRITERIA

The admissions procedure includes a file evaluation. There are no interviews.

ADDITIONAL REQUIREMENTS AND CONSIDERATIONS

Program of Study
Animal/Veterinary Experience
References
Employment History
Personal Statement
Extracurricular Activities
Entrance Requirements

To view our prerequisite courses for admission to the UGA College of Veterinary Medicine please visit our website at vet.uga.edu/admissions/requirements.

Required undergraduate GPA: cumulative GPA of 3.00 or greater on a 4.00 scale or a combined score on the GRE verbal and quantitative sections of 308 or higher.

Is a Bachelor's Degree Required? no

Is this an International School? no

ESTIMATED TUITION

Estimated Tuition Resident: approx. $19,436

Estimated Tuition Contract: approx. $19,436

Estimated Tuition Non-Resident: $48,516

AVAILABLE SEATS

Resident: 80

Contract: 19

Non-Resident: 15

TEST REQUIREMENTS

Standardized examinations: Graduate Record Examination (GRE) general test (including the analytical writing portion) must be completed within the 5 years immediately preceding the deadline for receipt.

VMCAS Participation: full

Accepts International Students? yes

ADDITIONAL INFORMATION

Combined DVM-graduate degree programs are available:

DVM-MPH Veterinarians in Public Health

DVM/PhD Veterinary Medical Scientist Training Program

Application Deadline: 9/17/2018

VMCAS Application Deadline: 9/17/2018

UNIVERSITY OF ILLINOIS

Email Address: admissions@vetmed.illinois.edu
Website: vetmed.illinois.edu

SCHOOL DESCRIPTION

The University of Illinois is in Urbana-Champaign, a community of 100,000 people located 140 miles south of Chicago. It is served by airports in Champaign, Chicago, Indianapolis, and St. Louis, 3 interstate highways, bus, and rail. The twin cities and university make a pleasant community with easy access to all areas and facilities. The university has 45,000 students and more than 11,000 faculty and staff members. It is known for its high-quality academic programs and its exceptional resources and facilities. It is the first university to have established a division of student disability resources. The university library has the largest collection of any public university and ranks third among all U.S. academic libraries. The university also has outstanding cultural and sports facilities and activities. The College of Veterinary Medicine is located at the south edge of the campus. In addition to over 500 veterinary students, the college has about 100 graduate students plus a full complement of residents and interns. There are more than 100 full-time faculty with research interests in a variety of biomedical sciences and clinical areas. This research activity offers a broad variety of experiences for students. The college also offers students a dynamic, integrated core-elective curriculum to prepare for careers in almost any area of the profession.

> It is known for its high-quality academic programs and its exceptional resources and facilities.

APPLICATION INFORMATION

For specific application information (availability, deadlines, fees, and VMCAS participation), please refer to our website: http://vetmed.illinois.edu/education/doctor-veterinary-medicine-degree/admissions

Supplemental questions specific to the University of Illinois are required and may be obtained from the Illinois page of the VMCAS application.

International applications are considered, although there are obvious constraints regarding translation of grades. The TOEFL will be required of any successful applicant before matriculation. U.S. Visa constraints may also be restrictive for admission.

Residency implications: priority is given to approximately 70 Illinois residents and 60 non-Illinois residents per class.

SUMMARY OF ADMISSION PROCEDURES

VMCAS application deadline: Monday, September 17, 2018 at 12 Midnight Eastern Time

Informational program and required interviews: mid-February

Date acceptances mailed: late February-early March

National application acceptance date: April 15, 2019

School begins: August 26, 2019

Deposit (to hold place in class): $500 deposit required on acceptance. Please check the Illinois Admissions website for the most current information.

Course Description*	Number of Hours/Credits	Necessity
Biological Science (with laboratories)	8	Required
Chemical Sciences (with laboratories)	16	Required
Physics (with laboratories)	8	Required

*With a bachelor's degree completed before matriculation in veterinary school. Without a bachelor's degree, all above must be taken; additional prerequisites are required in English Composition (3 hrs), Speech/Communication (3 hrs), Humanities/Social Science (12 hrs); 12 hrs of junior/senior/graduate level science courses.

Deferments: considered on an individual basis by the Associate Dean for Academic and Student Affairs.

EVALUATION CRITERIA

A 3-part admission procedure is used. An academic evaluation and an application evaluation of veterinary, animal experience and personal qualities are followed by a personal interview.

Academic evaluation: GRE test scores; Illinois science GPA; cumulative GPA; rigor of academic preparation

Nonacademic evaluation: veterinary-related experience, animal-related experience, community involvement, leadership, citizenship, and letters of recommendation; interview

ENTRANCE REQUIREMENTS

Required undergraduate GPA: a minimum cumulative GPA of 2.75 and a minimum Illinois science GPA of 2.75 on a 4.00 scale are required. The average statistics for students passing Admissions Phase I in 2014 were 3.59 cumulative GPA, 3.44 science GPA, and 65% GRE composite percentile

AP credit policy: AP credit is allowed to meet the 8 s.h. physics prerequisite requirement if a student is awarded the full 8 s.h. AP credit is allowed for biology and chemistry if it is followed up by more advanced college-level courses in those science areas.

GRE test within two years of application. Refer to website for specific dates.

Is a Bachelor's Degree Required? no

Is this an International School? no

ESTIMATED TUITION/FEES

Estimated Tuition Resident: $27,578 plus fees

Estimated Tuition Contract: not applicable

Estimated Tuition Non-Resident: $49,402 plus fees

AVAILABLE SEATS

Resident: 70

Contract: 0

Non-Resident: 60

TEST REQUIREMENTS

Standardized examinations: Graduate Record Examination (GRE), general test, is required. Test must be taken by September 1, 2018 for the 2018/2019 admission cycle. Test dates must be between August 1, 2016 and September 1, 2018. Tests outside this window will not be acceptable.

VMCAS Participation: full

Accepts International Students? yes

ADDITIONAL INFORMATION

Combined DVM/PhD programs may be available.

DVM/MPH with concurrent enrollment at University of Illinois at Chicago School of Public Health are also available.

Application Deadline: 9/17/2018

PRE-VETERINARY PROFILE: MEGAN BRIGHT

Current School Name
Arkansas State University

What type of veterinary medicine are you interested in pursuing, and why?
I am interested in pursuing large and small animal veterinary medicine. I am especially interested in working with farm animals and horses, as growing up on a beef cattle farm and in a rural community made me aware of the increased need for large animal veterinarians.

What is/was your major during undergraduate school?
My major was animal science with a pre-veterinary emphasis.

What are your short-term and long-term goals?
My short-term goals are to gain veterinary and animal-related experience during college breaks, begin studying for the GRE, and focus on doing well in all my classes. My long-term goals are to form a relationship with my veterinarian, become a more well-rounded individual, and pursue an internship with the USDA or a zoo.

What are you doing as an applicant/pre-vet to prepare for veterinary school?
I am currently working to gain as much veterinary and animal experience as possible by shadowing a local veterinarian, helping out at the humane society, and volunteering at a hippotherapy clinic. I have been working as an undergraduate research assistant at Arkansas Biosciences Institute for the past year in order to gain research experience. I am constantly setting short- and long-term goals while also researching the application process and requirements for veterinary school.

What extracurricular activities are you involved in currently?
I am involved in the Animal Science Club (combination of Pre-Vet Club, Equine Club, and Production and Management), Phi Beta Lambda, Honors College Association, Delta Tau Alpha, and intramural sports at Arkansas State University.

How old were you when you first became interested in being a veterinarian?
I have wanted to become a veterinarian since the time I learned what a veterinarian was at a young age; I have never wanted to be or do anything else.

Please describe your various experiences in preparation for applying to veterinary school.
As a sophomore at Arkansas State University, I am working closely with my adviser to ensure I take the appropriate veterinary school prerequisites. I have also purchased the AAVMC Admission Requirements book so I can begin forming a timeline and gathering the appropriate materials for applying to veterinary school. I plan to begin studying for the GRE soon, and I am seeking advice from my professors and veterinarians about the application process.

What characteristics are you looking for in a veterinary school?
I am looking for a veterinary school that has a good comparative research program because it's what I am interested in. I look for faculty in pathology or lab animal medicine so that they could possibly be a mentor to me when I am a student. I also am looking for a school that has a lower tuition cost and is in an area where the cost of living is lower.

What advice do you have for other pre-veterinary students?
My advice is to study hard, form close relationships with your professors, and get involved in clubs and volunteer activities on campus. Find ways to stay motivated throughout the semester, and stay up to date on the prerequisites and various requirements for each veterinary school you are interested in attending. If this is something that you truly want to do, work hard, set goals, and, most importantly, never give up.

IOWA STATE UNIVERSITY

Email Address: cvmadmissions@iastate.edu
Website: www.vetmed.iastate.edu

IOWA STATE UNIVERSITY
College of Veterinary Medicine

SCHOOL DESCRIPTION

As the nation's first public veterinary school, Iowa State University's College of Veterinary Medicine takes pride in its heritage while shaping the future of veterinary professional practice, education, research, and service.

Fully accredited by the American Veterinary Medical Association, the College of Veterinary Medicine is dedicated to the enhancement of the health and well-being of animals and human beings. In order for the college to carry out its mission, it focuses on students within the Doctor of Veterinary Medicine program and various graduate programs in each of five academic departments: Biomedical Sciences, Veterinary Clinical Sciences, Veterinary Diagnostic and Production Animal Medicine, Veterinary Microbiology and Preventive Medicine, and Veterinary Pathology.

Iowa State University shapes the future of veterinary professional practice, education, research, and service.

In addition to its five academic departments, the Veterinary Medicine complex houses the state's Veterinary Diagnostic Laboratory, the Hixson-Lied Small Animal Hospital, Large Animal Hospital, Wildlife Care Center, Clinical Skills Laboratory, Center for Food Security and Public Health, Iowa Center of Advanced Neurotoxicity, and the Institute for International Cooperation in Animal Biologics. The college is also home to the Swine Medicine Education Center, the nation's only center dedicated to providing veterinary students and practitioners from around the world with training in swine health and production medicine.

The college offers combined advanced degree programs for concurrent DVM students including the Masters of Business Administration with Iowa State's College of Business and the Masters of Public Health with the University of Iowa's College of Public Health.

On a daily basis, Iowa State addresses the health of all animals including livestock, poultry, companion animals, equine, captive and free-ranging wildlife, exotic animals, and birds. Researchers in the college have a global impact on not only animal health, but human health and food safety.

APPLICATION INFORMATION

The most current application information (availability, deadlines, fees, VMCAS participation), may be found at: http://vetmed.iastate.edu/academics/prospective-students/admissions

Supplemental Application: A supplemental application is required. The supplemental becomes available in early May and the link can be found at: http://vetmed.iastate.edu/academics/prospective-students/admissions

Residency implications: priority is given to Iowa residents for approximately 60 positions. Iowa contracts on a year-to-year basis with North Dakota and South Dakota. Iowa also has a formal educational alliance with Nebraska. Remaining positions are available for residents of noncontract states or international students.

SUMMARY OF ADMISSIONS PROCEDURES

Application deadline: Monday, September 17, 2018 at 12 Midnight Eastern Time

Date acceptances mailed: approximately February 15

School begins: late August

Deposit (to hold place in class): $500.00

Deferments: considered on a case-by-case basis

PREREQUISITES FOR ADMISSION

Course Description	Number of Hours/Credits	Necessity
General chemistry (1 year series w/lab)	7	Required
Organic chemistry (1 year series w/lab)	7	Required
Biochemistry	3	Required
Biology (1 year series w/labs)	8	Required
Genetics (Upper level Mendelian and molecular)	3	Required
Mammalian anatomy and/or physiology	3	Required
Oral communication (interpersonal, group or public speaking)	3	Required
English composition	6	Required
Social Science/Humanities	8	Required
Physics (Physics 1 - first semester of a 2 semester series with mechanics)	4	Required
Electives	8	Required

EVALUATION CRITERIA

The admission procedure consists of a review of each candidate's application and qualifications:
1. Academic factors include grades, test scores, and courseload.
2. Nonacademic factors include essays, experience, recommendations, and leadership and personal development activities.
3. Interviews are not conducted.

ENTRANCE REQUIREMENTS

Required undergraduate GPA: the minimum GPA required is 2.50 on a 4.00 scale. The most recent entering class had a mean GPA of 3.55.

AP credit policy: must be documented by original scores submitted to the university, and must meet the university's minimum requirement in the appropriate subject area. CLEP (College-Level Examination Program) credits accepted only for the arts, humanities, and social sciences.

Course completion deadline: It is preferred that prerequisite science courses be completed by the end of the fall term the year the applicant applies, and these must be completed with a C (2.0) or better to fulfill the requirement. However, up to 2 prerequisite science courses may be taken the spring term prior to matriculation. All other prerequisites must be completed by the end of the spring term prior to matriculation with a C (2.0) or better.

Pending courses may not be completed the summer prior to matriculation. Pass-not pass grades are not acceptable.

Is a Bachelor's Degree Required? no

Is this an International School? no

ESTIMATED TUITION

2018-2019 Tuition Resident: $24,500

Estimated Tuition Contract: Varies by contract

2018-2019 Tuition Non-Resident: $52,500

AVAILABLE SEATS

Resident (approximate): 60
Contract: 36
Non-Resident (approximate): 60

TEST REQUIREMENTS

Standardized examinations: Graduate Record Examination (GRE), general test, is required. Either the new Revised GRE or the previous GRE will be accepted, but the scores must either go directly from GRE to VMCAS or to Iowa State University College of Veterinary Medicine (code 6315). For the most current GRE submission information, please see the VMCAS instructions.

VMCAS Participation: full

Accepts International Students? yes

KANSAS STATE UNIVERSITY

Email Address: admit@vet.k-state.edu
Website: www.vet.k-state.edu

SCHOOL DESCRIPTION

Kansas State University in Manhattan, Kansas, is located 125 miles west of Kansas City near Interstate 70. With a population of about 70,000 including KSU, Manhattan is in an area surrounded by many historical points of interest in a rich agricultural area of north central Kansas. Recreational activities abound in Manhattan and the surrounding area with fishing, boating, camping, and hunting among the favorites. Sporting events, theater, concerts, and excellent parks contribute to the many activities available. Kansans enjoy the four seasons, each of which brings its own special activities and events.

> The College of Veterinary Medicine is located on 80 acres just north of the main campus in 3 connected buildings.

Kansas State University is on a beautiful 664-acre campus. The College of Veterinary Medicine opened in 1905. It is located on 80 acres just north of the main campus in 3 connected buildings.

APPLICATION INFORMATION

For specific application information (availability, deadlines, fees, and VMCAS participation), please refer to the contact information listed above.

Supplemental Application: Available at http://www.vet.k-state.edu/admissions/apply/ between May 11 and September 15.

Contract tuition: resident tuition

Resident seats: approximately 45

Nonresident seats: approximately 62

Contract seats: 5 with North Dakota

Residency implications: to be eligible to be in the Kansas pool of applicants, the applicant must be a Kansas resident for tuition purposes at the time of application. International applicants are considered. Kansas has a contract for students from North Dakota.

SUMMARY OF ADMISSION PROCEDURES

Timetable

VMCAS application deadline: Monday, September 17, 2018 at 12 Midnight Eastern Time

Kansas State University supplemental application deadline: postmarked by Monday, September 17, 2018

Kansas residents: mid-December interviews scheduled

Nonresident: early January interviews scheduled

North Dakota: February interviews scheduled

Date acceptances mailed: within 6 weeks after interview

School begins: mid-August

Deposit (to hold place in class): $500.00

Deferments: may be considered by Admissions Committee for extraordinary circumstances.

EVALUATION CRITERIA

An admission procedure is used including evaluation of science grades, evaluation of all 3 GRE scores, assessment of the application and narrative, and a personal interview.

PREREQUISITES FOR ADMISSION

Course Description	Number of Hours/Credits	Necessity
Expository Writing I and II	6	Required
Public Speaking	2	Required
Chemistry I and II	8	Required
General Organic Chemistry w/lab	5	Required
General Biochemistry	3	Required
Physics I and II	8	Required
Principles of Biology or General Zoology	4	Required
Microbiology w/lab	4	Required
Genetics	3	Required
Social Sciences and/or Humanities	12	Required
Electives	9	Required

30%: Prerequisite science GPA

30%: GRE test scores

40%: Interview score including:

    References

    Animal/veterinary experience

    Professionalism

    Problem solving

    Career awareness

    Leadership

ENTRANCE REQUIREMENTS

Prerequisites for Admission: Science courses must have been taken within six years of the date of enrollment in the professional program.

Required undergraduate GPA: the minimum required GPA to qualify for an interview is 2.80 on a 4.00 scale in both the prerequisite courses and the last 45 semester hours of undergraduate work. The most recent entering class had a mean prerequisite science GPA of 3.50.

AP credit policy: must appear on official college transcripts and be equivalent to the appropriate college-level coursework.

Course completion deadline: prerequisite courses must be completed by the end of the spring term of the year in which admission is sought.

Standardized examinations: Graduate Record Examination (GRE), general test, is required of all applicants. Scores are required to be reported by September 17.

ADDITIONAL REQUIREMENTS AND CONSIDERATIONS

Animal/veterinary work experience and knowledge

Employment record

3 evaluations required by nonfamily members: one veterinarian, one academic or preprofessional advisor, one professor or other professional.

Is a Bachelor's Degree Required? no

Is this an International School? no

ESTIMATED TUITION

Estimated Tuition Resident: $25,000

Estimated Tuition Contract: $25,000

Estimated Tuition Non-Resident: $55,000

AVAILABLE SEATS

Resident: 45-50

Contract: 5

Non-Resident: about 62

TEST REQUIREMENTS

Graduate Record Examination (GRE), general test

VMCAS Participation: full

Accepts International Students? yes

ADDITIONAL INFORMATION

Dual-Degree Programs

Combined DVM-graduate degree programs are available.

Combined DVM-MPH degree programs are available.

Early Admission Program

The Veterinary Scholars Early Admission Program is designed for those students having a genuine desire to enter the veterinary profession who attend Kansas State University with an ACT score of 29 or greater or an equivalent SAT score and who complete a successful interview during the fall semester of their freshman undergraduate year.

Application Deadline: 9/17/2018

LINCOLN MEMORIAL UNIVERSITY

Email Address: veterinaryadmissions@LMUnet.edu
Website: vetmed.lmunet.edu

LMU
Lincoln Memorial University

SCHOOL DESCRIPTION

Lincoln Memorial University (LMU) is an accredited, nonprofit university founded in 1897 through Abraham Lincoln's desire to provide an outstanding university for the people of Appalachia. The LMU main campus is located in Harrogate, Tennessee, beautifully situated at the foot of the historic Cumberland Gap and occupies more than 1,000 wooded acres with modern educational facilities that include classrooms and laboratories equipped with smart technology. Preclinical courses are taught at both the main Harrogate campus and at the DeBusk Veterinary Teaching Center (DVTC), utilizing state-of-the-art technology and clinical facilities about 15 minutes away from main campus in Ewing, Virginia.

> Hands-on animal and clinical skills-based experiences start in the first semester.

The goal of our innovative curriculum is to produce confident, competent, practice-ready veterinarians by emphasizing clinical and professional skills. All students receive a well-rounded education in small animal medicine, bovine and equine medicine as well as exposure to avian and exotic animal medicine.

Features of the LMU-CVM program:
- Hands-on animal and clinical or professional skills-based experiences start in the first semester and continuing throughout the entire curriculum.
- The large animal component of the DVTC provides a working farm environment with a large cattle and horse herd.
- Clinical Year Hybrid Distributive Education program prepares students by providing experience working in both primary care and specialty private practice environments. Students have flexibility through clinical electives to focus on the facets of veterinary medicine that interest them the most such as small animal, equine, or exotics.
- Veterinary research opportunities offer students valuable experience in this important facet of the profession. A diverse range of opportunities are available at LMU-CVM and with our partnership with the University of Kentucky.
- Case simulation labs teach professional and communication skills in an exam room environment with standardized patients in case scenarios.
- Students, staff, and faculty serve the health and wellness needs of people, animals, and the environment in Appalachia and beyond with an emphasis on the One Health approach.
- Our Shelter Outreach to the Appalachian Region (SOAR) program provides small animal spays and neuters for the Appalachian region while providing valuable learning expertise for veterinary students.

Outside of classes, LMU-CVM students have the opportunity to participate in student clubs and activities. LMU is centrally located between Knoxville, TN, and Lexington, KY, two major cities that offer many cultural and recreational opportunities. The Cumberland Gap National Park is a favorite location for students to hike, run, bicycle, and relax between classes.

PREREQUISITES FOR ADMISSION

Course Requirements	Semester Hours	Quarter hours
General Biology with lab	8	12
Genetics[1]	3	4
Biochemistry	3	4
Upper Division Science Electives (300 level or higher)[2]	8	12
Organic Chemistry with lab	6	9
General Chemistry with lab	6	12
Physics	3	4
English	3	4
Social and Behavioral Sciences	3	4

[1] Animal breeding/reproduction courses must be approved by LMU-CVM
[2] Upper Division coursework (300 level or higher) including Anatomy, Cell Biology, Immunology, Microbiology, Molecular Biology, Physiology, Virology

APPLICATION INFORMATION

A complete application includes: VMCAS application, LMU-CVM supplemental application, and GRE scores. Late or incomplete applications will not be considered.

For more admissions details, please visit our website.

SUMMARY OF ADMISSIONS PROCEDURE

Timetable

Application materials due: Monday, September 17, 2018 at 12 Midnight Eastern Time

On-campus Interviews: September–February

Notification of decision: March

Deposit (to hold place in class): $1,250.00

Orientation/Classes Begin: early August

EVALUATION CRITERIA

Each completed application will receive a holistic review based on both academic and non-academic factors. Some considerations include:
- Overall GPA, Science GPA, GPA in last 2 years of study
- GRE Scores
- Leadership skills evidenced by participation in student and community organizations
- Well-rounded life experience that demonstrates a judicious balance of academic achievement, community service, and personal interests
- Experience in and knowledge of the veterinary profession
- Written communication skills as seen in a personal statement
- Letters of recommendation submitted via VMCAS

ENTRANCE REQUIREMENTS

Required undergraduate GPA: Applicants must have a cumulative GPA of at least 2.8 on a 4.00 scale. Students who don't meet the minimum GPA requirement, who have demonstrated a commitment to academic excellence (GPA > 3.2) in the last 2 years of study (45 semester hours) may be considered on a case-by-case basis.

Prerequisite completion: All prerequisite courses must be completed with grade of a C- or higher by the end of the Spring 2018 semester. All science prerequisites must have been completed in the last 10 years, or after August 2007.

AP credit policy: AP courses are accepted if they are specifically listed on an official college transcript and are equivalent to the appropriate college-level coursework.

Is a Bachelor's Degree Required? no

Is this an International School? yes

ESTIMATED TUITION

Tuition: $46,250 (subject to change)

As a nonprofit institution, tuition is the same for all LMU-CVM students, regardless of state residency.

AVAILABLE SEATS

Class size: 115

As a nonprofit institution, LMU does not have separate resident and nonresident seats.

TEST REQUIREMENTS

The Graduate Record Examination (GRE), general test, is required and scores are due by September 17. Exams taken prior to August 2014 will not be accepted. Applicants should schedule the GRE at least 30 days prior to the deadline.

Additional requirements: All applicants are required to complete the LMU-CVM Supplemental Application found on the LMU-CVM website.

VMCAS Participation: full

Accepts International Students? yes

ADDITIONAL INFORMATION

Application deadline: 9/17/2018

Further details about the application process and the LMU-CVM program can be found at: vetmed.lmunet.edu.

Current School Name
University of Georgia

Why do you want to be a veterinarian?
I want to progress in my public health career while making meaningful contributions to the field of epidemiology and One Health as a whole. My background in field epidemiology and zoonotic and vectorborne disease make DVM the perfect degree to achieve my goals. Some of my greatest role models and closest colleagues/friends are public health veterinarians—I am lucky to know them and I believe they are incredibly important contributors to the field!

What are your short-term and long-term goals?
In the next 3.5 years, while I'm in vet school, I plan to find opportunities to keep working in field epidemiology during breaks and as a part of elective courses when possible. I want to make the most of my time in the program and learn as much as I can prior to graduation. In the long-term, I hope to take a position as a medical epidemiologist post-graduation either at the state health department, Centers for Disease Control and Prevention (CDC), or with an international organization.

What did you do as an applicant to prepare for applying to veterinary school?
I had been out of college for quite a while, so I took a couple of upper level biology/chemistry courses at a local college to get back into the swing of classroom learning and to show the admissions committee that I could still excel in that setting. I was working full time so I had open communication with my workplace about applying—they were very supportive and helped to work around my class schedule for courses. I also looked at all of the schools of veterinary medicine and learning about each (cost, strengths, focus, requirements for admission, etc.). I tried to get some varied experiences, as well; most of my veterinary experience was in research, so I found a shelter that I could volunteer at every other Sunday for a vaccine clinic.

What advice would you give to applicants or those considering applying to veterinary school?
Find a way to make yourself stand out! Aside from that, make sure you research any school you are applying to—it can give you insight into what they are looking for in an applicant. People often apply to multiple schools, which is smart, but it's more efficient (and probably more effective) to only apply to schools you've had time to really look at, make sure you meet the requirements for, and that "make sense" for you as an applicant. I would always recommend considering the schools that are most cost-effective for you as a student. Finally, be open-minded going into school, not knowing for sure what you want to do after. It can be an amazing opportunity to find what you love and are passionate about. However, before you apply/start, be 100% sure that whatever you want to do requires a DVM degree.

What helped make the transition to veterinary school easier for you?
I am a lot older than many of my classmates and come from years of working full time, so I'll be honest that the transition into vet school was difficult for me in a lot of ways. I struggled at first to find my place, but being flexible and proactive really helped me to work through that. Although vet school is your "life," you are not defined by it. Make time for yourself and keep up relationships with old friends. Also, if your school doesn't take the initiative to help you find researchers or opportunities in your area of interest, don't be afraid to search the directory and reach out to people. You never know what connections you'll make and what opportunities might come from them! Finally, try to stay positive and make friends within your class.

What is your advice on student debt?
I strongly advise prioritizing the school(s) cheapest for you. You can create opportunities anywhere and work with people in other fields or at other schools during breaks—there are veterinary scholars programs at a lot of schools that welcome applicants from other schools. However, that debt will be with you for a long time and will impact your quality of life. Actively trying to minimize the debt you need to take out now will help give you a better quality of life after school.

What are you most excited about learning in veterinary school?
Everything! (I mean, almost everything ;)). I am excited to continue to progress through the curriculum to apply the building blocks we are learning now to more tangible situations.

LOUISIANA STATE UNIVERSITY

Email Address: svmadmissions@lsu.edu
Website: www.lsu.edu/vetmed

SCHOOL DESCRIPTION

The Louisiana State University campus is located in Baton Rouge, which has a population of more than 500,000 and is a major industrial city, a thriving port, and the state's capital. Since it is located on the Mississippi River, Baton Rouge was a target for domination by Spanish, French, and English settlers. The city bears the influence of all three cultures and offers a range of choices in everything from food to architectural design. Geographically, Baton Rouge is the center of south Louisiana's main cultural and recreational attractions. Equally distant from New Orleans and the fabled Cajun bayou country, there is an abundance of cultural and outdoor recreational activities. South Louisiana has a balmy climate that encourages lush vegetation and comfortable temperatures year round.

> Geographically, Baton Rouge is the center of south Louisiana's main cultural and recreational attractions.

The campus encompasses more than 2,000 acres in the southern part of Baton Rouge and is bordered on the west by the Mississippi River. The Veterinary Medicine Building, occupied in 1978, houses the academic departments, the veterinary library, the Louisiana Animal Disease Diagnostic Laboratory, the Wildlife Hospital of Louisiana, and the Veterinary Teaching Hospital. The school is fully accredited by the American Veterinary Medical Association.

APPLICATION INFORMATION

For specific application information (availability, deadlines, fees, and VMCAS participation), please refer to the LSU SVM admissions website at www.lsu.edu/vetmed/dvm_admissions.

Residency implications: The LSU SVM accepts 60-65 in-state residents and has approximately 9 seats reserved for AR contract students. The remaining 40-60 seats are offered to non-resident students. International students can be accepted as long as prerequisite courses have been taken in North America or coursework is certified as to U.S. equivalence.

SUMMARY OF ADMISSION PROCEDURES

Timetable

Suggested last date to take GRE: August 15

VMCAS application deadline: Monday, September 17, 2018 at 12 Midnight Eastern Time

Supplemental application deadline: All LSU SVM-specific questions in the VMCAS application must be completed as per the VMCAS instructions and by the VMCAS application deadline. (There is no supplemental application for the LSU SVM outside of the VMCAS application.)

LSU SVM application processing fee ($90) deadline: October 1

GRE score submission deadline: October 1 (use VMCAS-specific School Code - 2281, listed as Louisiana State University-VMCAS)

Date interviews are held: February*

Date acceptances mailed: late February/early March

School begins: early to mid-August

PREREQUISITES FOR ADMISSION

Course Description	Number of Hours/Credits	Necessity
General Biology	8	Required
Microbiology (w/lab)	4	Required
Physics	6	Required
General Chemistry	8	Required
Organic chemistry	3	Required
Biochemistry	3	Required
English Composition	6	Required
Speech Communication	3	Required
Mathematics	5	Required
Electives	20	Required

*Interview invitations are extended to a select number of Louisiana, Arkansas, and out of state applicants as determined by the LSU SVM Admissions Committee.

Deposit (to hold place in class): $500.00 for non-residents only

Deferments: considered on a case-by-case basis

EVALUATION CRITERIA

The approximate components of the evaluation scoring are:

Objective evaluation:
    GPA required courses: 29%
    GPA last 45 hours: 18%
    Test scores: 18%

Subjective evaluation:
    Animal/veterinary experience, references (min. of 3 required, one by a veterinarian), essay, knowledge of profession, etc.: 15%
    Personal interview: 10%
    Committee evaluation: 10%

ENTRANCE REQUIREMENTS

Required undergraduate GPA: the minimum acceptable GPA for required coursework is 3.00 on a 4.00 scale. The mean GPA of the most recent entering class at the time of acceptance was 3.80.

AP credit policy: must appear on official college transcripts and be equivalent to the appropriate college-level coursework.

Is a Bachelor's Degree Required? no

Is this an International School? no

ESTIMATED ANNUAL TUITION

Estimated Tuition Resident: $27,000

Estimated Tuition Contract: $33,500

Estimated Tuition Non-Resident: $56,900

AVAILABLE SEATS

Resident: 60-65

Contract: 9

Non-Resident: 20-40

TEST REQUIREMENTS

Standardized examinations: The GRE revised General Test is required. The scores must be received no later than October 1. Note: All applicants must take the GRE revised General Test.

VMCAS Participation: full

Accepts International Students? The LSU SVM will accept international students as long as all prerequisite coursework has been completed at an accredited institution within the United States or Canada. Foreign coursework is not accepted in fulfillment of the course prerequisites unless certified as to U.S. equivalence.

ADDITIONAL INFORMATION

Application Deadline: 9/17/2018

MICHIGAN STATE UNIVERSITY

Email Address: admiss@cvm.msu.edu
Website: http://www.cvm.msu.edu

SCHOOL DESCRIPTION

Michigan State University's campus is bordered by the city of East Lansing, which offers sidewalk cafes, restaurants, shops, and convenient mass transit. The campus is traversed by the Red Cedar River and has many miles of bike paths and walkways. This park-like setting provides an ideal venue in which MSU's 48,906 students may enjoy outdoor concerts and plays, canoeing, and cross-country skiing. The campus is located in East Lansing, three miles east of Michigan's capitol in Lansing. It sits on a 5,200-acre campus with 2,100 acres in existing or planned development. There are 532 buildings which include 103 academic buildings.

> Michigan State University is a national leader in state-of-the-art technology and facilities.

TOP DISTINCTIONS

U.S. News & World Report ranks MSU 33rd among the nation's public universities; 75% among the world's top 100 universities; first in the nation for 22 years for graduate programs in elementary; and secondary education. First in the nation for graduate programs in nuclear physics, organizational psychology, and rehabilitation counseling. One of the top 70 universities in the world.

The College of Veterinary Medicine is fortunate to have an outstanding faculty, all of whom hold the doctor of veterinary medicine degree and/or the doctor of philosophy degree. Nearly all of the specialty boards recognized by the American Veterinary Medical Association are represented on the faculty. Many of these faculty members are leaders in their fields, both nationally and internationally.

Today, the college includes four biomedical science departments—microbiology and molecular genetics, pathobiology and diagnostic investigation, pharmacology and toxicology, and physiology; two clinical departments—large-animal clinical sciences and small-animal clinical sciences; two service units—the Veterinary Diagnostic Laboratory for Population and Animal Health; and several research centers.

Michigan State has a long-standing commitment to equal opportunity, affirmative action, and multiculturalism. The College of Veterinary Medicine has attained national recognition for its leadership in programs for the encouragement of underrepresented groups at the preprofessional, professional, and advanced studies levels, as well as for increased diversity in its faculty.

APPLICATION INFORMATION

For specific application information (pre-requisite science courses, deadlines, and VMCAS participation), please refer to our website: http://cvm.msu.edu

Residency implications: priority is given to Michigan residents. Up to 37 positions are filled with nonresident and international applicants.

SUMMARY OF ADMISSION PROCEDURES

VMCAS application deadline: Monday, September 17, 2018 at 12 Midnight Eastern Time

Electronic evaluations to VMCAS: Monday, September 17, 2018 at 12 Midnight Eastern Time.

Submit transcripts from *all* colleges attended to VMCAS by Monday, September 17, 2018, *including*

Course Description	Number of Hours/Credits	Necessity
English Composition	3	Required
Social and Behavioral Sciences	6	Required
Humanities	6	Required
General Inorganic Chemistry (with Laboratory)	3	Required
Organic Chemistry (with laboratory)	6	Required
Biochemistry (upper division)	3	Required
General Biology (with laboratory)	6	Required
College Algebra and Trigonometry	3	Required
College Physics (with laboratory)	8	Required
Upper Level Biology Elective Course	3	Required

For the most accurate information about the prerequisites, please contact the Office of Admissions at admiss@cvm.msu.edu

colleges where you took courses that transfer to your main institution.

International transcripts must be evaluated by World Education Services (WES) and submitted to VMCAS. It is recommended that transcript(s) be submitted to the translation service at least one month prior to the deadline of Monday, September 17, 2018.

Non-refundable deposit (to hold place in class): (non-refundable) $500.00 for residents; $1,000.00 for non-residents

Deferments are rare.

ENTRANCE REQUIREMENTS

Required undergraduate GPA: The minimum required GPA for science prerequisite courses is 3.0 and for the last three semesters GPA is 3.0. The means for the most recent entering class were a science prerequisite GPA of 3.59 and a last three semester GPA of 3.77. The last three semester GPA includes a minimum of 36 credits for undergraduate students and a minimum of 18 credits for a graduate student. (NOTE: The last 3-semester GPA can include more than three semesters if the minimum of 36 credits (or 18 if graduate work) was not completed in just three semesters.)

AP credit policy: AP credit(s) must appear on an official transcript and be equivalent to appropriate college-level coursework.

Is a Bachelor's Degree Required? no

Is this an International School? no

ESTIMATED TUITION

Estimated Tuition Resident: $30,400

Estimated Tuition Contract: $0

Estimated Tuition Non-Resident: $56,512

AVAILABLE SEATS

Resident: 78

Contract: 0

Non-Resident: 37

TEST REQUIREMENTS

Standardized examinations: International applicants who are non-native speakers of English and who do not hold a bachelor's degree from a US institution must take a test of English as a second language. Options are the TOEFL iBT, the IELTS, or the CAEL.

VMCAS Participation: full

Accepts International Students? yes

ADDITIONAL REQUIREMENTS AND CONSIDERATIONS

Evaluation of written application (including animal/veterinary/research/extracurricular/employment/volunteer experiences)

Letters of recommendation (3 submitted by Monday, September 17, 2018, at 12 Midnight Eastern Time through VMCAS; 1 must be completed by a veterinarian)

Multiple Mini Interview or MMI

Acceptance deadline is Monday, April 15, 2019

2015-2016 ADMISSIONS SUMMARY

Number of Applicants: 1,199

Number of New Entrants

Resident: 78

Non-Resident/International: 37

Total: 115

EXPENSES AND FEES (ESTIMATED AS OF 2017)

Resident: $30,400

Non-resident: $56,512

EARLY ADMISSION PROGRAM

The Veterinary Scholars Admission Program has been established by the College of Veterinary Medicine in cooperation with the Honors College at Michigan State University. This program provides admission opportunity for students who wish to enter the four year professional veterinary medicine degree program after earning a bachelor's degree. The bachelor's degree program must include advanced and enriched coursework representing scholarly interest and achivments. Enrollment at MSU and membership in the Honors College are required to be eligible for this option. For information on Honors College membership, contact: Honors College, 105 Eustace-Hall, 468 E. Circle Drive, Michigan State University, East Lansing, MI 48824; telephone (517) 355-2326; or visit their website at http://honorscollege.msu.edu.

PRODUCTION MEDICINE PATHWAY

The Production Medicine Scholars Pathway has been established by the College of Veterinary Medicine in cooperation with the department of Animal Sciences at Michigan State University. This pathway is available to MSU Animal Science students who complete, in addition to the minimum pre-veterinary medicine requirements, a bachelor's degree in Animal Sciences with a concentration in production animal medicine. The concentration is designed to prepare students for a career in herd based, agricultural veterinary practice. The pathway provides an early admission option for Michigan State University students planing to earn a baccalaureate degree in Animal Science with a concentration in production medicine. Successful applicants must have a strong academic and non-academic credentials, a demonstrated interest in food animal production medicine and agricultural veterinary medicine. Additional information about the pathway may be obtained from 1250 Anthony Hall, 474 S. Shaw Lane, Department of Animal Science, Michigan State University, East Lansing, MI 48824 or visit the website: http://www.ans.msu.edu.

DUAL DEGREE PROGRAMS

Combined DVM-MPH degree program available

Combined online DVM/MS in Food Safety available

Application Deadline: 9/17/2018, midnight EST

MIDWESTERN UNIVERSITY

Email Address: admissaz@midwestern.edu
Website: www.midwestern.edu

SCHOOL DESCRIPTION

The Midwestern University College of Veterinary Medicine (MWU-CVM) presents to its students a four year program leading to the Doctor of Veterinary Medicine (DVM) degree. The first 8 quarters are a mix of classroom lectures, laboratories, simulation lab exercises with virtual clients and patients, and small group, student-centered learning experiences. Hands-on live animal contact begins in the first quarter and continues throughout the program. Quarters 9-13 involve diverse clinical training, both on campus (about 85%) and at external sites (about 15%). Three new buildings, including a 111,000 square foot small animal Veterinary Teaching Hospital and a roughly 36,000 square foot large animal/pathology facility, insure our students will begin their careers in state-of-the-art surroundings.

> Three new buildings insure MWU-CVM students will begin their careers in state-of-the-art surroundings.

In October, 2014, the American Veterinary Medical Association Council on Education (AVMA-COE) extended provisional accreditation to the College. This notification indicates that the University and College submitted a plan which successfully met the 11 standards required by the AVMA to become accredited. The program will be eligible for full accreditation in 2018, upon graduation of the first class.

APPLICATION INFORMATION

The CVM utilizes the Veterinary Medical College Application Service (VMCAS). The VMCAS application is available online at www.aavmc.org. The VMCAS application cycle opens in June of each year. The official VMCAS application deadline is September 17, 2018 at 12 Midnight Eastern Time. Midwestern accepts direct applications after the close of the VMCAS cycle. Requests for withdrawing an application must be submitted in writing. In accordance with the Association of American Veterinary Medical Colleges acceptance deadline policy, students are not required to accept or reject an offer of admission until April 15th. Students may accept or reject earlier if so inclined. If a signed letter accepting admission and the required deposit are not received by April 15th, the offer of admission may be withdrawn.

SUMMARY OF ADMISSION PROCEDURES

Students seeking admission to the CVM must submit the following documented evidence:
1. Completion of prerequisite coursework or plans to complete the coursework prior to matriculation. (Confirmed by official transcripts)
   a. Minimum science AND minimum total cumulative GPA of 2.75 on a 4.00 scale.
   b. No grade lower than a C in any course will be accepted for credit. (Pass/fail and satisfactory/ unsatisfactory grading is not acceptable in prerequisite science courses.)
2. Completion of a minimum of 240 hours (6 weeks) of veterinary, health sciences, animal or biomedical

PREREQUISITES FOR ADMISSION

Course Description	Number of Hours/Credits	Necessity
Biology	8	Required
Biochemistry	3	Required
General Chemistry	8	Required
Organic Chemistry with Lab	8	Required
Mathematics	6	Required
Physics with Lab	4	Required
English Composition	6	Required
Science Electives	8	Required

A minimum of 64 total semester hours/96 quarter hours is required.

research experience. Students with additional hours of work experience will present a stronger case for admission.

3. Competitive scores on the GRE General Test taken no more than 5 years prior to the planned enrollment year.

4. Three letters of recommendation.
   a. At least one of the letters must be from a veterinarian.
   b. The other letters can be from other veterinarians, or from pre-veterinary or science professors, or from someone who can testify to the integrity and ethical standards of the applicant.
   c. Letters written by family members are not acceptable.
   d. Letters must be submitted by evaluators. Letters submitted by students are not accepted by the Office of Admissions.

5. Although not required, a Bachelor's degree will make a candidate more competitive.

ENTRANCE REQUIREMENTS

1. Demonstrate an understanding of the veterinary medical profession.
2. Demonstrate service orientation through community service or extracurricular activities.
3. Have a proper motivation for and commitment to the veterinary profession as demonstrated by previous salaried work, volunteer work, or other life experiences.
4. Possess the oral and written communication skills necessary to interact with patients, clients, and colleagues.

5. Pass the Midwestern University criminal background check.
6. Abide by Midwestern University's Drug-Free Workplace and Substance Abuse Policy.
7. Meet the Technical Standards for the College (see below).

Is a Bachelor's Degree Required? no

Is this an International School? no

ESTIMATED TUITION

Estimated Tuition Resident: $59,454

Estimated Tuition Contract: $59,454

Estimated Tuition Non-Resident: $59,454

AVAILABLE SEATS

100

TEST REQUIREMENTS

Graduate Record Exam

VMCAS Participation: full

Accepts International Students? yes

ADDITIONAL INFORMATION

Science electives include cell biology, physiology, microbiology, genetics, animal nutrition, etc.

Minimum of 64 total semester hours/96 quarter hours

Application Deadline: 9/17/2018

UNIVERSITY OF MINNESOTA

Email Address: dvminfo@umn.edu
Website: https://www.vetmed.umn.edu/education/
dvm/admissions

UNIVERSITY OF MINNESOTA

College of Veterinary Medicine

SCHOOL DESCRIPTION

The University of Minnesota College of Veterinary Medicine prepares future leaders in companion animal, food animal, and public health practice, as well as research and education. University of Minnesota students benefit from one of the largest teaching hospitals in the country, as well as world renowned faculty in zoonotic diseases, comparative medicine, and population systems. The College offers state-of-the-art facilities, including the Veterinary Medical Center, Leatherdale Equine Center, and the Raptor Center, which in 1988 became the world's first facility designed specifically for birds of prey. Off-site facilities include farms throughout Minnesota and around the world.

> Students gain hands-on experience throughout the entire program in clinical and professional skills courses.

The College of Veterinary Medicine is located on the 540-acre St. Paul campus. Students enjoy a small, intimate campus atmosphere of approximately 3,000 students while benefiting from the numerous amenities available within one of the nation's largest university systems.

The Twin Cities of Minneapolis and St. Paul have a combined population of approximately 2.5 million people and represents one of the largest metropolitan areas where a veterinary college is located. The Twin Cities is the cultural center for the region, abundant with outdoor recreational opportunities, and is repeatedly cited as one of the most livable metropolitan areas in the nation.

In 2013-14, the DVM program underwent a complete curriculum revision. During the first three years of the DVM program, students focus on the study of the normal animal, the pathogenesis of diseases and the prevention, alleviation and clinical therapy of diseases. Students gain hands-on experience throughout the entire program in clinical and professional skills courses.

The program concludes with thirteen months of clinical rotations in the Veterinary Medical Center, during which time students learn methods of veterinary care and develop skills needed for professional practice. Students can choose from over 70 rotation offerings. The fourth year includes up to ten weeks of externship experiences at off-campus sites of the student's choice.

APPLICATION INFORMATION

Application requirements include a complete VMCAS application, three electronic letters of reference submitted through VMCAS, official transcripts submitted through VMCAS, GRE examination scores, and an $85 application processing fee. The University of Minnesota College of Veterinary Medicine does not utilize a supplemental application.

The application, transcripts, and references are due to VMCAS by their respective deadlines.

All other application materials are due to the College by the application deadline of September 17, 2018 at 12 Midnight Eastern Time. For more application information, please visit https://www.vetmed.umn.edu/education/dvm/admissions.

Residency implications: first priority is given to residents of Minnesota and residents of states with which a reciprocity or contract agreement exists (North Dakota and South Dakota). Residents of other states are encour-

PREREQUISITES FOR ADMISSION

Course Description	Number of Hours/Credits
English (2 courses)	6
Algebra, Pre-Calculus, or Calculus	3
General Chemistry w/ Labs (2 courses, plus 2 labs)	6
Organic Chemistry	3
Biochemistry	3
General Biology w/ Lab	3
Zoology w/ Lab	3
Genetics	3
Microbiology w/ Lab	3
Physics (2 courses)	6
Liberal Education (3 courses)	9
Statistics	3

aged to apply. International applicants should contact the Admissions Office for additional information. The University of Minnesota will accept 105 students into the program each year. Approximately 53 of the 105 seats are reserved for resident/reciprocity eligible applicants. Approximately 52 seats are held for non-resident applicants.

SUMMARY OF ADMISSION PROCEDURES

Timetable

VMCAS application deadline: Monday, September 17, 2018 at 12 Midnight Eastern Time

Date acceptances communicated: mid- to late February

School begins: last week of August

Deposit (to hold place in class): $500.00

Deferments: can be requested for extenuating circumstances that warrant a 1-year delay in admission. Requests to defer submitted after July 15 will not be considered.

EVALUATION CRITERIA

Objective measures of educational background

• GPA in prerequisite coursework

• GPA in most recent 45-semester credits

• GRE Test scores

Behavioral interviews

Subjective measures of personal experience

• Employment record

• Extracurricular and/or community service activities

• Leadership abilities

• References

• Maturity/reliability

• Animal/veterinary knowledge, experience, and interest

2017-2018 ADMISSIONS SUMMARY

Number of Number of Applicants / New Entrants

Resident: 156/52 admitted

Non-Resident: 655/52 admitted

Total: 811/104 admitted

The figures for new entrants include students taking delayed admission from the previous year.

*Includes residents of North and South Dakota

EXPENSES FOR THE 2017-2018 ACADEMIC YEAR

Tuition and fees

Residents: $31,700*

Nonresidents: $56,972*

*This includes all tuition, fees, and two semesters of health insurance costs (approximately $2,100). Health insurance is mandatory; students can petition out of insurance costs if proof of personal coverage is provided.

Students from Minnesota and South Dakota pay resident tuition rates. Students from North Dakota can apply to the state of North Dakota for tuition support through the Professional Student Exchange Program (PSEP). Approved North Dakota students pay resident tuition rates. North Dakota students not approved pay non-resident tuition rates. Students from all other states or international locations pay non-resident tuition rates.

Students may apply for residency after one year of enrollment.

ENTRANCE REQUIREMENTS

All prerequisites must be graded at a C- or better. Math and science prerequisites courses must be recent within ten years of the application deadline.

Liberal education requirements: A minimum of three courses (9 credits) designated as liberal education by the applicant's undergraduate institution attended.

Required undergraduate GPA: 2.75 minimum GPA required for prerequisite GPA and last-45 semester credit GPA. The class of 2021 had a mean GPA of 3.60 (on a 4.00 scale) for required courses and 3.68 for the last 60 quarter-hour or 45 semester-hour credits of coursework prior to admission.

AP credit policy: must appear on official college transcripts and be equivalent to the appropriate college-level coursework.

Course completion deadline: prerequisite courses must be completed by the end of the spring term (not later than June 15) of the academic year in which application is made. No more than five prerequisite science and math courses may be pending completion during the fall and spring semesters of the application cycle. Science laboratory courses are not included in the count of five.

Standardized examinations: Graduate Record Examination (GRE), general test, is required. Results must be received by the College by the application deadline. The mean combined score for the verbal and quantitative sections of the GRE for the class of 2021 was 312. When scheduling your exam, confirm that your test date will allow enough time for results to be delivered by the application deadline of September 17. Send test results to institution code 6904.

Is a Bachelor's Degree Required? no

Is this an International School? no

ESTIMATED TUITION

Estimated Tuition Resident: $31,700

Estimated Tuition Contract: n/a

Estimated Tuition Non-Resident: $56,972

AVAILABLE SEATS

Resident: 53

Contract: n/a

Non-Resident: 52

TEST REQUIREMENTS

Graduate Record Exam

VMCAS Participation: full

Accepts International Students? yes

ADDITIONAL INFORMATION

Application Deadline: 9/17/2018

PRE-VETERINARY PROFILE: TYLER BRZOZOWSKI

Current School Name
Wilkes University

What type of veterinary medicine are you interested in pursuing, and why?
I plan to be a large animal veterinarian. Small animal medicine is also important to me and will be one of my focuses. I have been dealing with large animals for quite some time now, and I have grown to love the science behind them.

What is/was your major during undergraduate school?
My major is biology/pre-vet.

What are your short-term and long-term goals?
My short-term goals are to gain admittance into vet school—my dream school is Cornell University. I am also trying to gain as much experience as possible before then. My long-term goals are to graduate from vet school and get proper licensing for my veterinary practice. I then plan to specialize in large animal medicine and work with small animals on the side.

What are you doing as an applicant/pre-vet to prepare for veterinary school?
I am preparing myself for vet school by exposing myself to multiple areas of the veterinary field, as well as multiple types of animals (large, small, exotic, etc.), and by being a well-rounded individual in my school and public lives. Experience and grades are most important to me, and I volunteer at various veterinary clinics. I also work at Pocono Downs Racetrack for standard-bred harness racing, where I am practicing sample collections and handling skills.

What extracurricular activities are you involved in currently?
I am Vice President of the Hudson Model Railroad Club located in Hudson, Pennsylvania. At Wilkes University, I am Vice President of our Pre-Vet Club. I enjoy hunting and fishing as well as being out in nature hiking or just relaxing. I enjoy horseback riding and I plan to start an equestrian sport such as polo.

How old were you when you first became interested in being a veterinarian?
I was about eight years old when I finally decided that veterinary medicine was what I wanted to do for the rest of my life.

Please describe your various experiences in preparation for applying to veterinary school.
Growing up I had two dogs, a bearded dragon, and two cats. My sister has a horse farm that I regularly visit (it's like my second home). I experienced all of the basics—most importantly, proper safety precautions. I also experienced horse training, dental procedures, farrier procedures, farm-calls, Xrays, euthanasia, sedation, and more. I have also volunteered at a local vet clinic, where I assisted with surgeries such as spays and neuters, exploratory surgeries, yearly checkups, euthanasia, sample handling, and patient and client welfare. I currently work at Pocono Downs Racetrack for harness racing. There I assist the state veterinarian with pre-race blood-gas testing, as well as post-race urine and blood sampling. I also have a lot of one-on-one contact with people.

What characteristics are you looking for in a veterinary school?
I am looking for a nice community of veterinarian scientists. I am not particularly sure of my preferred learning environment (traditional vs. case-based) but I am very adaptable to change and I am intrigued by challenges. I am a hands-on type person and I am hoping for even more exposure to the veterinary field.

What advice do you have for other pre-veterinary students?
Follow your dreams and don't ever let anyone pull you down. I have had numerous people try to talk me out of this profession and even at times say I can't do it. I respond by saying, "Say I can't, so I can show you I can." You should also get tons of experience with various types of animals. This profession is not simply about "loving animals." That matters, but the true meaning of this profession (at least to me) is having a passion for healing animals and for the science and medicine behind the healing. Also, broaden your horizon! Don't be afraid to experiment, and, most importantly, don't be afraid to fail! We learn from our mistakes and will always make more of them. Be sure to excel in your education. You might do poorly on some exams, and you might begin to question yourself and lose confidence, but allow yourself to realize the potential outcome of your life—veterinary medicine.

MISSISSIPPI STATE UNIVERSITY

Email Address: MSU-CVMAdmissions@cvm.msstate.edu
Website: www.cvm.msstate.edu

SCHOOL DESCRIPTION

Starkville is home to 22,000 MSU students and their Bulldogs. Starkville is located in northeast central Mississippi and has a population of 24,000. Being a land-grant university, MSU is green and beautifully landscaped. The university includes 9 farms scattered throughout the state. The College of Veterinary Medicine (the Wise Center) was completed in 1982. The college includes 620 rooms on 8 acres, or 360,000 square feet, under one roof.

> The curriculum of the MSU-CVM is divided into 2 phases: Phase 1 or Pre-clinical and Phase 2 or Clinical.

The curriculum of the MSU-CVM is divided into 2 phases: Phase 1 or Pre-clinical (freshman and sophomore years) and Phase 2 or Clinical (junior and senior years).

Year 1 uses foundation courses to expose the student to important medical concepts and address multidisciplinary problems.

Year 2 is devoted to the study of clinical diseases and abnormalities of animal species. Surgery labs begin in the second year.

Year 3 is comprised of clinical rotations in the College's Animal Health Center, and elective courses.

Year 4 includes core rotations in internal medicine and ICU, large animal ambulatory, neurology, ophthalmology, and the Jackson Emergency/Referral Clinic.

The remainder of the fourth year is largely experiential and offers the student the opportunity to select among approved experiences in advanced clinical rotations, elective courses, and/or externships. The first 3 years of the curriculum are 9-10 months in length, while the fourth year is 12 months.

APPLICATION INFORMATION

For specific application information (availability, deadlines, fees, and VMCAS participation), please refer to the contact information listed above.

Residency implications: Mississippi State accepts 40 Mississippi residents, 5 contract students from South Carolina, 7 contract students from West Virginia, and 43 non-resident applicants.

SUMMARY OF ADMISSION PROCEDURES

Timetable

VMCAS application deadline: Monday, September 17, 2018 at 12 Midnight Eastern Time

GRE General Exam scores and supplemental application deadline: The GRE is not required.

Date interviews are held: late January or February

Date acceptances mailed: February

First-year classes begin: early July

Deposit (to hold place in class): $500.00

Deferments: requests are considered on an individual basis

PREREQUISITES FOR ADMISSION

Course Description	Number of Hours/Credits	Necessity
English Composition and/or Academic Writing	6	Required
Speech or Technical Writing	3	Required
Mathematics (College Algebra or higher)	6	Required
General Biology and accompanying labs	8*	Required
Microbiology with laboratory	4	Required
General Chemistry and accompanying labs	8*	Required
Organic Chemistry and accompanying labs	8*	Required
Biochemistry	3	Required
Physics (may be Trig-based)	6	Required
Advanced (upper-level) science electives	12	Required
Humanities, fine arts, social sciences and behavioral electives	15	Required

* indicates requirement of a minimum 6 hours of lecture and 2 hours of laboratory

EVALUATION CRITERIA

Grades (minimum competitive GPAs are typically 3.3-3.4)

Quality of academic program

Test scores

Animal/veterinary experience

Participation in extra-curricular and community service activities and outside employment

Leadership and interpersonal skills

References (3 required; one must be from a veterinarian)

Personal statement

Interview of applicants selected on basis of academic and non-academic criteria

ENTRANCE REQUIREMENTS

Required undergraduate GPA: a minimum overall GPA of 2.8 on a 4.0 scale. The minimum GPA must be maintained throughout the application process. The class of 2021 has an average undergraduate GPA of 3.62.

At time of application and throughout the application period, no grade lower than a C- s acceptable in any required course. Remediated and repeated courses must be completed before the application is submitted.

AP credit policy: must appear on official college transcripts and be equivalent to the appropriate college-level coursework.

Is a Bachelor's Degree Required? no

Is this an International School? no

2017-2018 TUITION AND FEES

Estimated Tuition Resident: $26,200

Estimated Tuition Contract: $26,200

Estimated Tuition Non-Resident: $47,400

AVAILABLE SEATS

Resident: 40

Contract: 12

Non-Resident: 43

TEST REQUIREMENTS

Standardized examinations: Graduate Record Exam (GRE), general test, is not required.

VMCAS Participation: full

Accepts International Students? yes

ADDITIONAL INFORMATION

DVM-PhD Program

The mission of the MSU-CVM DVM-PhD program is to prepare exceptional students for careers as veterinary scientists to meet the nation's critical needs in animal and human health research. It is the intent of the MSU-CVM DVM-PhD program to provide the full rigor of training from the DVM and PhD degrees as if they were pursued separately. The program is designed to integrate the research and clinical training programs so that students will experience a logical progression and level of responsibility throughout the program. It is also the intent of the program to provide a system of moral and financial support for the students who have committed to it.

Please contact Dr. Mark Lawrence, Associate Dean for Research and Graduate Programs, at lawrence@cvm.msstate.edu for more information.

MSU-CVM EARLY ENTRY PROGRAM

The Early Entry Program is a unique program of the College of Veterinary Medicine (CVM) that allows high-achieving high school seniors to earn pre-acceptance (early, pre-approved acceptance) into the CVM.

Students who have an interest in veterinary medicine and meet application requirements during high school may apply for the Early Entry Program. If a student is accepted into this program, he/she begins undergraduate work at MSU after high school graduation, and completes the first three to four years of prerequisite courses, while also working toward completion of a bachelor's degree. After the student has completed all course requirements for the College of Veterinary Medicine, has remained in good standing, and has taken the GRE General Exam, he/she matriculates into the CVM as a pre-accepted student. The student does not make further application to the CVM.

Students applying for this program must have the following qualifications:

1. ACT composite score of 27 (SAT score of 1820 on new SAT); and
2. High school grade average of 90 (3.6 on a 4.0 scale)

In addition, the Early Entry Program Admissions Committee considers animal and veterinary experience, work experience, leadership qualities, and nontechnical skills and aptitudes (character, community service, etc.) as described in the applicant's written application to the Early Entry Program, and in the applicant's Letters of Recommendation (provided in the application).

Twenty-five positions are available each year. We normally receive 70 to 80 applications. Both Mississippi and out-of-state students are eligible for the program.

Applications for the Early Entry Program are available by October 1 each year, and are due for return by January 5. Applicants are notified of acceptance status by early February.

Applications are available online from October 1 through December 31. Please see the following website for the application and important information: http://www.cvm.msstate.edu/academics/early_entry_program.html

Application Deadline: 1/5/2019

UNIVERSITY OF MISSOURI

Email Address: seayk@missouri.edu
Website: cvm.missouri.edu/prospective.htm

SCHOOL DESCRIPTION

The University of Missouri is located among rolling forested hills north of the famous Lake of the Ozarks. Columbia is noted for its high quality of life and low cost of living and is consistently rated among the best cities to live in by Money Magazine. The city abounds with walking trails, 3,000 acres of state park lands, federal forests, and wildlife refuges. Columbia is located between Kansas City and St. Louis-cities that have major-league sports teams and other big-city recreational amenities. Columbia itself offers SEC Conference football, basketball, baseball and other sports. It boasts a 71,168-seat stadium, several 18-hole golf courses, and other indoor and outdoor recreation facilities. Our location near a metropolitan area provides a strong primary and referral small animal case load. Columbia's proximity to rural central Missouri results in an exceptional food animal and equine case load.

> The unique curriculum gives students 2 years of undiluted clinical experience before graduation.

MU, a major research university with 33,000 students, consists of 18 schools and colleges located on a 1,262-acre campus. The College of Veterinary Medicine is noted for its unique curriculum that gives students nearly 2 years of clinical experience before graduation as opposed to the traditional 1-1.5 years. Students benefit from exposure to specialty medical areas such as clinical cardiology, neurology, orthopedics, ophthalmology, and oncology. Students also gain experience with advanced equipment such as a linear accelerator for treatment of cancer, MRI, state-of-the-art ultrasonography, extensive endoscopy equipment, cold lasers, a surgery room C-arm for radiography during surgical procedures, and others. MU is unique in having a medical school, nursing school, school of health-related professions, state cancer research center, the life sciences center, and department of animal science on the same campus, thus enhancing teaching, research, and clinical services.

APPLICATION INFORMATION

All applicants must apply through VMCAS and submit our Supplemental Application. For specific application information (availability, deadlines, fees, and VMCAS participation), please refer to the contact information listed above.

Residency implications: sixty seats are given to Missouri and sixty to non-residents. A total of 120 seats awarded each year. U.S. citizenship or permanent residency is required. Allows non-residents to gain residency after completing first year.

SUMMARY OF ADMISSION PROCEDURES

Mid-May 2018: VMCAS Application Opens.

August 1, 2018: Transcripts due to VMCAS.

VMCAS application, GRE scores, and all letters of reference due: September 17, 2018 at 12 Midnight Eastern Time

Supplemental Missouri application due: September 18, 2018

Early January: Out-of-state interviews held. Must appear in person if invited.

February–March: Missouri interviews held.

PREREQUISITES FOR ADMISSION

Course Description	Number of Hours/Credits	Necessity
English or Communication	6	Required
College algebra or higher	3	Required
Physics (complete sequence)	5	Required
Biological Science - not AS courses	10	Required
Humanities/Social Sciences	10	Required
Biochemistry with organic pre-req	3	Required
Electives	10	Required

Mid-April: Decisions mailed.

Late August: Orientation and school begins.

ENTRANCE REQUIREMENTS

Required undergraduate GPA: Applicants must have a cumulative GPA of 3.00 or more on a 4.00 scale. The most recent entering class had a mean GPA of 3.77 at the time of acceptance.

AP credit policy: must appear on official college transcript and be equivalent to the appropriate college-level coursework.

Is a Bachelor's Degree Required? no

Is this an International School? no

ESTIMATED TUITION

Estimated Tuition Resident: $25,696.16

Estimated Tuition Contract: pending

Estimated Tuition Non-Resident: $60,980.96

AVAILABLE SEATS

Resident: 60

Contract: pending

Non-Resident: 60

TEST REQUIREMENTS

Standardized examinations: Graduate Record Examination (GRE) general test, including the analytical writing portion, must be completed within the last 3 years. A score of 285 (verbal and quantitative added together) and a 1.5 on the analytical is required. (Test must be taken after September 15, 2015 and submitted to VMCAS by September 17, 2018)

VMCAS Participation: full

Accepts International Students? no

ADDITIONAL INFORMATION

Application Deadline: 9/17/2018

NORTH CAROLINA STATE UNIVERSITY

Email Address: dvminformation@ncsu.edu
Website: www.cvm.ncsu.edu

NC STATE UNIVERSITY | College of Veterinary Medicine

SCHOOL DESCRIPTION

The North Carolina State University College of Veterinary Medicine consistently ranks as one of the leading veterinary educational programs in North America. Located in the state capital of Raleigh, the campus resides in one of the most desirable areas to live and work. The region is home to one of the nation's leading research parks and provides students with opportunities for collaborations in biotechnology, biomedicine, and environmental health with industry and government researchers, clinical trial companies, and other academic colleagues.

> The College of Veterinary Medicine has 160 faculty members and a capacity for 400 veterinary medical students.

With delightful mountains and beaches nearby, a mild climate, and a thriving local economy, the 250-acre Centennial Biomedical Campus, anchored by the College of Veterinary Medicine, is a magnet for students, faculty, and project partners alike.

Featuring 160 faculty members and a capacity for 400 veterinary medical students, the college also offers training for interns, residents, and graduate students. The campus includes a state-of-the-art teaching hospital, classrooms, a working farm, research and teaching laboratories, and a variety of additional amenities. The Randall B. Terry, Jr., Companion Animal Veterinary Medical Center offers cutting-edge technologies for imaging, cardiac care, cancer treatment, and internal medicine and surgery, and handles more than 30,000 referral cases a year. In addition, the educational model has been fully revamped with an eye on the future, equipping students for success in private practice, industry, government, and academia, with emphasis on teamwork, client interactions, and communication skills.

Classroom spaces throughout the college have been substantially remodeled and expanded in the past three years, including a communications training center and a psychomotor skills laboratory, as well as a remodeled original companion-animal hospital as a first-opinion clinic. The college remains a leader in affordability for prospective students and continues to emphasize diversity as a critical part of its overall mission. It also features an excellent student-faculty ratio and offers a multitude of hands-on educational experiences.

The NC State Veterinary Medicine community enhances animal and human health and well-being through the education and advanced training of veterinarians and comparative biomedical scientists. The community is dedicated to providing leadership in veterinary care, biomedical discovery, and societal engagement that addresses complex global issues facing animal, human, and environmental health. It raises the bar for teaching, healing, and scientific discovery in the 21st century.

APPLICATION INFORMATION

For specific application information (availability, deadlines, fees, and VMCAS participation), please refer to the contact information listed above.

Residency implications: priority is given to North Carolina residents. NOTE: The college increased its incoming class size from 80 to 100 starting with the 2012 admissions cycle. The current slot allocation is 80 resi-

PREREQUISITES FOR ADMISSION

Course Description	Number of Hours/Credits	Necessity
Animal Nutrition	3	Required
Biochemistry	3	Required
Biology	4	Required
Chemistry, General	8	Required
Chemistry, Organic	8	Required
Composition, Public Speaking or Communications	6	Required
Humanities and Social Sciences	6	Required
Microbiology	4	Required
Physics	8	Required
Statistics	3	Required
Genetics	4	Required

dent and 20 non-resident slots. Non-resident admits are permitted to apply for residency for tuition purposes after the first 12 months in the program.

SUMMARY OF ADMISSION PROCEDURES

VMCAS application deadline: Monday, September 17, 2018 at 12 Midnight Eastern Time

NC State Supplemental application deadline: Monday, September 17, 2018 at 1:00 PM Eastern Time

Date acceptances mailed: no later than April 1

School begins: August

Deposit (to hold place in class): $250.00

Deferments: are considered for 1 year only, subject to approval by the Assistant Dean.

EVALUATION CRITERIA

Selection for admission is a 2-phase process.

Phase 1-Objective criteria:

Required course GPA: 3.0 Resident, 3.4 Nonresident

Cumulative GPA: 3.0 Resident, 3.4 Nonresident

Last 45 credit hour GPA: 3.0 Resident, 3.4 Nonresident

GRE test score

Supplemental Application

Phase 2-Subjective criteria:

1. Veterinary Experience
2. Animal Experience
3. Educational Experience
4. Evaluation Forms/Recommendations
5. Personal Statement
6. Diversity
7. Extracurricular and Community Activities

ENTRANCE REQUIREMENTS

AP credit policy: must appear on official college transcripts with course name and credit hours and be equivalent to the appropriate college-level coursework.

Is a Bachelor's Degree Required? no

Is this an International School? yes

ESTIMATED TUITION

Estimated Tuition Resident: $18,970

Estimated Tuition Contract: $0

Estimated Tuition Non-Resident: $45,160

AVAILABLE SEATS

Resident: 80

Contract: 0

Non-Resident: 20

TEST REQUIREMENTS

Standardized examinations: Graduate Record Examination (GRE), general test, is required. The scores must be received by the September 17 application deadline. There is no deadline to take the GRE.

VMCAS Participation: full

Accepts International Students? yes

ADDITIONAL INFORMATION

Application Deadline: 9/17/2018

THE OHIO STATE UNIVERSITY

Email Address: dvmprospective@osu.edu
Website: www.vet.osu.edu/admissions

THE OHIO STATE UNIVERSITY

COLLEGE OF VETERINARY MEDICINE

SCHOOL DESCRIPTION

The Ohio State University is located in Columbus, the state's capital and the nation's 15th largest city. Columbus has been rated the 7th best city in the nation for cost of living (Forbes Magazine) and one of the country's top-10 places to live (Money). Columbus offers all the cultural perks you would expect from a major metropolitan area including the #1 zoo in the country, according to the USA Travel Guide.

The Ohio State University was founded in 1870 and is one of the nation's leading academic centers, consistently ranks as Ohio's best, and one of the nation's top-20 public universities. The campus consists of thousands of acres, hundreds of buildings, more than 15,000 faculty and staff, and more than 56,000 students.

The Veterinary Medical Center includes a Hospital for Companion Animals, Food Animal, and the Galbreath Equine Center. The patient load is one of the highest in the country and farmlands can be accessed 10 miles from campus. The Veterinary Medicine Academic Building has nearly 10,000 square feet of space and includes research labs, classrooms, a library, computer lab, and academic offices. The Ohio State University College of Veterinary Medicine is ranked fifth in the nation among veterinary schools according to U.S. News & World Report's "Best Graduate Schools."

The Ohio State College of Veterinary Medicine is part of one of the largest and most comprehensive

> The college is part of one of the largest and most comprehensive health sciences centers in the country.

health sciences centers in the country that includes dentistry, medicine, nursing, optometry, pharmacy, public health, and veterinary medicine.

APPLICATION INFORMATION

For specific application information (availability, deadlines, fees, and VMCAS participation), please refer to the contact information listed above.

Residency implications: applicants from all states will be considered. In-state and out-of-state applicants are given equal consideration. We accept the top 162 students. We do accept international applicants.

SUMMARY OF ADMISSION PROCEDURES

VMCAS application deadline: Monday, September 17, 2018 at 12 Midnight Eastern Time

Date interviews are held: January-February

Date acceptances mailed: February-March

School begins: late August

Deposit (to hold place in class): $25.00 for residents; $300.00 (non-refundable fee) for non-resident applicants

Deferments: not considered

EVALUATION CRITERIA

1. Objective Score = Overall GPA + Science GPA + Last 30 hours (GPA)

2. Application Review which include:

• Veterinary and animal experience (depth & diversity of experience)

PREREQUISITES FOR ADMISSION

Course Description	Semester Hours (hours may vary)	Notes
Biochemistry*	4	If Biochemistry is taught as a 2-part sequence, both parts are required. Lab is not required.
Microbiology*	4	Lab is required.
Physiology**	5	Physiology can be awarded for a single intro-level Human or Animal Physiology course covering all systems, or a two part combined Anatomy & Physiology sequence (2 qtrs or 2 sems, Must have both courses to fulfill). Lab is not required.
Public Speaking (Communication)	3	Basics of public speaking & critical thinking. This should be a public speaking course.
Science Electives	35	Includes, but not limited to: Biology, chemistry, anatomy, immunology, cell biology, molecular genetics, animal science, ecology, environmental science or other science courses.
Humanities/Social Science Electives	16	Includes, but not limited to: History, economics, anthropology, psychology, art, music, literature, languages, writing, and ethics.

* = Capstone Courses

**Physiology course work must be a comprehensive, intermediate systems physiology series. Required systems include musculoskeletal, neurology, urinary/renal, endocrine, reproductive, digestive, cardiovascular, and respiratory.

Science electives can include courses that are prerequisites for the capstone courses (e.g. biology, general and organic chemistry, etc.).

The number of hours provided is a guideline. In assessing course content for equivalency, actual hours may vary for your institution. In some cases a multiple course series may be needed to fulfill prerequisite coursework. If you are unsure of whether or not a course will be accepted to fulfill a prerequisite, please contact us at prospective@cvm.osu.edu.

Capstone courses - Biochemistry, Microbiology, Physiology, and Communication - must be completed with (1) a grade of C or better in each course, (2) a 3.0 (B) average among the courses, and (3) no more than one C between any of the four courses.

   •If any of the capstone courses are taken as a multiple-part series, this rule will apply to each part as an individual course.

There may be additional courses that your school requires as prerequisites to the above courses. These additional courses can be used toward the elective requirements.

ADVANCED PLACEMENT

To receive credit for AP courses, they must be listed on official transcripts from a college or university you have attended.

- Community/Volunteer Service, Work and Leadership Experience

- Overall evaluation of application which includes review of personal state and letters of recommendations (Three are required at least one must be a veterinarian)

*Objective Score + Application Review Score determines if a student qualifies for an interview

3. In person interview - traditional interview style with at least two people.

ENTRANCE REQUIREMENTS

Required undergraduate GPA: the minimum GPA to be considered is 3.0 on a 4.0 scale. The most recent entering class had a mean overall GPA of 3.68 and a science GPA of 3.54. Science GPA is evaluated as well as last 30 semester or quarter hours.

AP credit policy: AP credit given if course is listed on official transcript.

Is a Bachelor's Degree Required? no

Is this an International School? no

COURSE COMPLETION DEADLINE

All of the prerequisite courses must be completed by the end of the summer term preceding the autumn term when you would start vet school. You do not have to have all the prerequisites completed before applying.

ESTIMATED TUITION

Estimated Tuition Resident: $31,160

Estimated Tuition Contract: $0

Estimated Tuition Non-Resident: $70,091 (first year)

Tuition is subject to change.

*For tuition purposes, nonresident students can apply for residency after completing their first year at the Ohio State University.

AVAILABLE SEATS

Accept 162 students.

Resident: Up to 100

Contract: 0

Non-Resident: Up to 80

TEST REQUIREMENTS

No test requirements.

VMCAS Participation: full

Accepts International Students? yes

ADDITIONAL INFORMATION

Application Deadline: 9/17/2018

VETERINARIAN PROFILE: MARTA POWERS

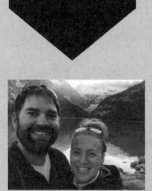

YEAR OF GRADUATION
2011

PLACE OF EMPLOYMENT
Anoka Equine Veterinary Services

What is your favorite aspect of being a veterinarian?
Being a veterinarian can be a challenge; however, it is filled with beautiful moments when you help patients and the humans who love them.

What type of veterinary medicine do you practice?
I practice almost exclusively equine veterinary medicine with a focus on reproduction and neonatology.

Where did you attend veterinary school?
University of Minnesota College of Veterinary Medicine.

How long have you been practicing as a veterinarian?
Since my graduation in 2011.

What advice do you have for those considering a career in veterinary medicine?
Veterinary medicine offers many diverse opportunities. Students interested in pursuing a career veterinary This career path is wonderful; however, it is not without its frustrating moments. I strongly recommend people considering a career in veterinary medicine shadow and have one-on-one time with current veterinarians. Talk about the good and the bad. Talk about school debt, and think seriously about what you learn.

What challenges have you faced while practicing veterinary medicine?
Veterinary medicine requires good mental aptitude to be able to manage a variety of challenges and There have been many challenges: school debt, work-life balance, moral and ethical challenges in relation to clients and colleagues, self- doubt, and so forth.

OKLAHOMA STATE UNIVERSITY

Email Address: dvm@okstate.edu
Website: www.cvhs.okstate.edu

SCHOOL DESCRIPTION

Oklahoma State University is located in Stillwater, which has a population of about 50,000. Stillwater is in north central Oklahoma about 65 miles from Oklahoma City and 69 miles from Tulsa. The campus is exceptionally beautiful, with modified Georgian-style architecture in the new buildings. It encompasses 840 acres and more than 60 major academic buildings.

Three major buildings form the veterinary medicine complex. The oldest, McElroy Hall, houses the William E. Brock Memorial Library and Learning Center, as well as classrooms and laboratories. The Boren Veterinary Medical Teaching Hospital provides modern facilities for both academic and clinical instruction. Completing the triad is the Oklahoma Animal Disease Diagnostic Laboratory, which provides teaching resources for students in the professional curriculum and diagnostic services to Oklahoma agriculture and industry. The College of Veterinary Medicine is fully accredited by the American Veterinary Medical Association. Faculty members in the three academic departments share responsibility for the curriculum. These departments are Veterinary Clinical Sciences, Veterinary Pathobiology, and Physiological Sciences.

> Faculty members in the three OSU academic departments share responsibility for the curriculum.

APPLICATION INFORMATION

Residency implications: entering class size is 106, which includes 58 Oklahoma residents and 48 non-residents. A non-resident contract seat is available through AR.

SUMMARY OF ADMISSION PROCEDURES

Timetable

VMCAS application deadline: Monday, September 17, 2018 at 12 Midnight Eastern Time

Date interviews held: February

Date acceptances mailed: March

School begins: mid-August

Deposit (to hold place in class): resident, $100.00; non-resident, $500.00

EVALUATION CRITERIA

The admission procedure consists of evaluation of both academic and nonacademic criteria. The Admissions Committee considers all factors in the applicant's file, but the following are especially important: academic achievement; familiarity with the profession and sincerity of interest; recommendations; test scores; extracurricular activities; character, personality, and commitment for a career in veterinary medicine. The committee selects those applicants considered most capable of excelling as veterinary medical students and who possess the greatest potential for success in the veterinary medical profession.

PREREQUISITES FOR ADMISSION

Course Description	Minimum Number of Hours/Credits	Necessity
Animal Nutrition	3	Required
Biochemistry	3	Required
Biology/Zoology	8	Required
English, Speech, or Composition	9	Required
Genetics	3	Required
Humanities/Social Science	6	Required
Inorganic Chemistry	8	Required
Math (College Algebra - No Statistics)	3	Required
Microbiology	4	Required
Organic Chemistry (5-hour survey accepted)	8	Required
Physics 1 & 2	8	Required

Starting in the fall of 2019, statistics will be required for all applicants.

ENTRANCE REQUIREMENTS

Required undergraduate GPA: a minimum GPA of 2.8 (on a 4.0 scale) is required in prerequisite courses. The mean cumulative GPA of the 2017 entering class was 3.59.

AP credit policy: AP credit accepted if documented on college transcript.

Is a Bachelor's Degree Required? no

Is this an International School? no

ESTIMATED TUITION

Estimated Tuition Resident: $22,570 (tuition + fees for one full year)

Estimated Tuition Contract: $0

Estimated Tuition Non-Resident: $48,550 (tuition + fees for one full year)

AVAILABLE SEATS

Resident: 58

Contract: 0

Non-Resident: 48

TEST REQUIREMENTS

Standardized examinations: Graduate Record Examination (GRE), general test, is required. The class of 2021 had mean scores of 152 verbal, 151 quantitative, and analytical of 4.0. Scores must be sent to code 6558 by October 15.

VMCAS Participation: full

Accepts International Students? yes

ADDITIONAL INFORMATION

Application Deadline: 9/17/2018

OREGON STATE UNIVERSITY

Email Address: cvmadmissions@oregonstate.edu
Website: www.oregonstate.edu/vetmed

SCHOOL DESCRIPTION

Oregon State University is located in Corvallis, the heart of the Willamette Valley. Our climate is mild year-round, with ocean beaches less than an hour drive to the west and some of the best snow skiing in the Cascade Range a little over two hours to the east. Major metropolitan attractions can be found less than two hours away in Eugene, Salem and Portland. Corvallis has a population of approximately 55,000 and is a beautiful and friendly place to live and pursue your education.

> Hands-on education is an important aspect to how our students learn and develop knowledge of the profession.

The Oregon State University College of Veterinary Medicine has one of the smallest class sizes of the DVM programs in the U.S., admitting just 72 students per year. Hands-on education is an important aspect to how our students learn and develop their knowledge of the profession. Our partnership with the Oregon Humane Society provides an opportunity for students to continue acquiring skills and confidence in their ability to perform as professionals. Students at OSU work in state-of-the-art facilities alongside our world-class faculty, including specialists in cardiology, oncology, imaging, and rehabilitation. The individual attention our students get from faculty and hospital staff is, in part, why year after year nearly 100% percent of our students pass their board exams.

APPLICATION INFORMATION

All components of the Oregon State DVM application are due by September 17. No materials will be accepted after this date including transcripts and GRE scores.

SUMMARY OF ADMISSION PROCEDURES

Steps to apply for admission to Oregon State University College of Veterinary Medicine:

1. Begin the VMCAS application process
2. Request all transcripts be sent direct to VMCAS, they must be received by September 17, 2018.
   VMCAS Transcripts
   P O Box 9126
   Watertown, MA 02471
3. Submit GRE scores directly to VMCAS using ETS code 4565.
4. Complete VMCAS with electronic letters of recommendation
5. Complete Oregon State University supplemental application by September 17, 2018 at 12 Midnight Eastern Time.
6. Pay online supplemental application fee of $50.00

ENTRANCE REQUIREMENTS

All pre-requisites for OSU must be completed with a grade of C- or better.

Is a Bachelor's Degree Required? no

Is this an International School? yes

PREREQUISITES FOR ADMISSION

Course Description	Number of Hours/Credits	Necessity
General Biology I	3	Required
General Biology II	3	Required
Upper Division Biology w/ Lab	4	Required
Physics I	4	Required
Physics II	4	Required
General Chemistry I w/ Lab	4	Required
General Chemistry II w/ Lab	4	Required
Organic Chemistry I	3	Required
Biochemistry I	4	Required
Genetics	3	Required
Calculus or Algebra & Trig	4	Required
Statistics	3	Required
Physiology (Human or Animal)	3	Required
*English	4	Required
*Humanities or Social Sciences	8	Required
*Public Speaking	3	Required

*Please note that the General Education Requirements (English, Humanities, & Public Speaking) will be considered met if the applicant has earned a bachelor's degree by July 1 of the year in which they are accepted into the program.

ESTIMATED TUITION

Estimated Tuition Resident: $23,874

Estimated Tuition Contract: $23,874

Estimated Tuition Non-Resident: $46,029

AVAILABLE SEATS

Resident: 40

Non-Resident (including Contract positions): 32

TEST REQUIREMENTS

VMCAS Participation: full

Accepts International Students? yes

ADDITIONAL INFORMATION

Conversion for quarter credits of our pre-requisites is available on our website.

Application Deadline: 9/17/2018

UNIVERSITY OF PENNSYLVANIA

Email Address: admissions@vet.upenn.edu
Website: www.vet.upenn.edu

SCHOOL DESCRIPTION

The University of Pennsylvania is located in West Philadelphia. Philadelphia is a city with a strong cultural heritage. Independence National Park includes 1 square mile of historic Philadelphia next to the Delaware River. Included are Independence Hall, the Liberty Bell, and many fine examples of colonial architecture. Philadelphia also offers theaters, museums, sports, and outdoor recreation. The Philadelphia Zoo, first in the nation, houses more than 1,600 mammals, birds, reptiles, and amphibians.

> The School of Veterinary Medicine enjoys a close relationship with the Philadelphia zoo, first in the nation.

The School of Veterinary Medicine enjoys a close relationship with the zoo. The School of Veterinary Medicine was founded in 1884 and includes a hospital for small animals, classrooms, and research facilities in the city. The large-animal hospital and research facilities are located at the New Bolton Center, an 800-acre farm 40 miles west of Philadelphia. The first 2 years are spent on the main campus. Part of the third year may be spent at the New Bolton Center, and the fourth year is spent in rotation and on electives at varying campus locations. Off-campus electives are frequently permitted.

APPLICATION INFORMATION

For specific application information (availability, deadlines, fees, and VMCAS participation), please refer to the contact information listed above.

Residency implications: priority is given to Pennsylvania residents. The number of nonresident places is usually about 85, including international applicants.

2016–2017 admissions summary for the class of 2021:

	Number of Applicants	Number of Entrants
Resident	221	40
Non-Resident	935	75
Total	1,156	115

SUMMARY OF ADMISSION PROCEDURES

Timetable

VMCAS application deadline: Monday, September 17, 2018 at 12 Midnight Eastern Time

Supplemental application and fee deadline: September 17. For more information, visit: http://www.vet.upenn.edu/education/admissions/application-process

Date interviews are held: Fridays from early January until completion

Date acceptances mailed: within 14 days after interview

School begins: late August/early September

Deposit (to hold place in class): $500.00

Deferments: are considered on an individual basis.

EVALUATION CRITERIA

The seats are filled through a 2-part admission procedure, which includes a file review and personal interviews.

Grades

Test scores

PREREQUISITES FOR MATRICULATION	
Course Description	**Number of Hours/Credits**
English (including composition)	6
Physics (with lab)	8
Chemistry - General (with at least 1 lab)	8
Chemistry - Organic	4
Biology or Zoology (covering basic genetics & cell bio)	9
Biochem	3
Microbiology	3
Social sciences or humanities	6
Calculus & Statistics (Any Introductory Stats course)	6
Electives	37

Animal/veterinary experience

Interview

References

Essay

English skills (TOEFL)

File review: files are reviewed in late Fall by members of the admissions committee (including an alumni member), and decisions are made on whether or not to offer an interview.

Personal interviews: interviews are held on Fridays from early January until the class is filled. The number of interviews granted equals approximately 2 times the number of seats available.

Two personal interviews are conducted: (1) a formal interview with 1 faculty member or PennVet alumni member of the committee and a second faculty member or alum who is not a committee member; and (2) an informal interview with student committee members. Although students do not vote on acceptance, they have a significant part in the meeting following interviews.

ENTRANCE REQUIREMENTS

Required undergraduate GPA: no specific GPA. Applicants are evaluated comparatively. The mean cumulative GPA of the class admitted in 2017 was 3.58.

AP credit policy: must appear on official college transcripts and count toward degree.

Course completion deadline: Requirements do not need to be complete in order to apply.

ADDITIONAL REQUIREMENTS/CONSIDERATIONS

Animal/veterinary work experience: experience working with animals, direct veterinary work, or research experience is desired. Approximately 500-600 hours is recommended. Experience should be sufficient to convince the admissions committee of motivation, interest, and understanding.

Recommendations/evaluations: 3 required, one from an academic science source; and one from a veterinarian. The third is the choice of the applicant.

Extracurricular/community service activities: additional activities in this category can provide information important to the admissions committee.

Leadership: evidence of leadership abilities is desirable.

Is a Bachelor's Degree Required? no

Is this an International School? no

ESTIMATED TUITION

Estimated Tuition and Fees Resident: $43,310

Estimated Tuition and Fees Contract: Not Applicable

Estimated Tuition and Fees Non-Resident: $53,310

AVAILABLE SEATS

Resident: 40

Contract: Not Applicable

Non-Resident: 85

TEST REQUIREMENTS

Standardized examinations: Graduate Record Examination (GRE), general test, is required; the GRE Code for Pennvet is 2775. Test scores should be received no later than October 15.

VMCAS Participation: full

Accepts International Students? yes

ADDITIONAL INFORMATION

Dual-Degree Programs: Combined VMD graduate degree programs are available and include the VMD-PhD, the VMD-MPII, and the VMD-MBA.

Summer Program: Penn Vet offers a summer program for high school and college students. The Veterinary Exploration Through Science (VETS) program, now in its eighth year is a day program of one-week sessions designed for those who want a close-up look at veterinary medicine. For additional information, please visit our website at www.vet.upenn.edu/education/admissions/summer-vets-program or call 215-898-5434.

Application Deadline: 9/17/2018

PURDUE UNIVERSITY

Email Address: vetadmissions@purdue.edu
Website: www.vet.purdue.edu
Phone: 765-494-7893

INDIANA

SCHOOL DESCRIPTION

Purdue University is located in one of the largest metropolitan centers in northwestern Indiana. Greater Lafayette occupies a site on the Wabash River 65 miles northwest of Indianapolis and 126 miles southeast of Chicago. The combined population of the twin cities, Lafayette and West Lafayette, exceeds 100,000. The community offers an art museum, historical museum, 1,600 acres of public parks, and more than 60 churches of all major denominations.

> Purdue emphasizes the veterinary team approach, problem solving, and hands-on experiences.

Purdue ranks among the 25 largest colleges and universities in the nation. Students represent all 50 states and many foreign countries. Purdue University has the third highest enrollment of international students of any college in the United States. The Purdue University College of Veterinary Medicine strives to become the leading veterinary school for comprehensive education of the veterinary team and for discovery and engagement in selected areas of veterinary and comparative biomedical sciences. To better prepare individuals for veterinary medical careers in the twenty-first century, our curriculum emphasizes the veterinary team approach, problem-solving, and hands-on experiences.

APPLICATION INFORMATION

For specific application information, please refer to the contact information listed above.

Each veterinary class has 84 students. The class will be seated with approximately 50% residents and 50% nonresident students.

SUMMARY OF ADMISSION PROCEDURES

Timetable

VMCAS application deadline: Monday, September 17, 2018 at 12 Midnight Eastern Time

Date interviews are held: January

Date acceptances released: February

Classes begin: late August

Deposit (to hold place in class): $1,000.00 deposit for resident and nonresidents. Deposit applied to tuition after matriculation. Deposit are not refundable.

Deferments: request for deferments will be considered on a case-by-case basis.

EVALUATION CRITERIA

The admission process consists of:

A preliminary review based upon grade point indices and prerequisite course completion

An in-depth review of selected applicants

A personal interview by invitation is required

% Weight

Grades, overall academic performance - 55% weight (including academic rigor)

Animal, veterinary, research, and general work experiences, extracurricular activities, leadership, personal

PREREQUISITES FOR ADMISSION

Course Description	Semester(s)	Necessity
General (Inorganic) Chemistry with Lab I	1	Required
General (Inorganic) Chemistry with Lab II	1	Required
Organic Chemistry with Lab I	1	Required
Organic Chemistry with Lab II	1	Required
Biochemistry (upperlevel)	1	Required
General Biology with Lab I	1	Required
General Biology with Lab II	1	Required
Genetics	1	Required
Microbiology with Lab	1	Required
Animal Nutrition	1	Required
Physics with Lab I	1	Required
Physics with Lab II	1	Required
Statistics	1	Required
English Composition	1	Required
Communication	1	Required
Humanities	3	Required

statements, overall presentation of application materials, honors and awards, references, and interview - 45% weight

ENTRANCE REQUIREMENTS

Required undergraduate GPA: the mean cumulative GPA of the entering class in the fall of 2017 for resident students was 3.69 on a 4.00 scale and for non-resident students was 3.58 on a 4.00 scale. The minimum cumulative GPA required for consideration is 3.00 on a 4.00 scale.

AP credit policy: will be accepted if it appears on official college transcripts by subject area and is equivalent to the appropriate college-level coursework. Should your institution's official transcript not list the subject area, then you may submit an unofficial transcript with a letter explaining this and indicating which prerequisite courses are met by these credits.

Is a Bachelor's Degree Required? no

Is this an International School? no

ESTIMATED TUITION

Estimated Tuition Resident: $19,928

Estimated Tuition Contract: n/a

Estimated Tuition Non-Resident: $44,756

AVAILABLE SEATS

Resident: 42

Contract: 0

Non-Resident: 42

TEST REQUIREMENTS

Standardized examinations: none

VMCAS Participation: full

Accepts International Students? yes

ADDITIONAL INFORMATION:

Application Deadline: 9/17/2018

PRE-VETERINARY PROFILE: CHRIS CLARKSTON

Current School Name
Kansas State University

What type of veterinary medicine are you interested in pursuing, and why?
Many different aspects of veterinary medicine fascinate me. It is such a diverse and growing field that I have not decided which career path I want to take after vet school. Currently, I have a particular interest in infectious disease research and specialized animal health, such as dentistry or surgery. As an undergraduate, though, I have decided to keep an open mind about all potential career paths associated with a DVM degree.

What is/was your major during undergraduate school?
Microbiology.

What are your short-term and long-term goals?
The evident short-term goal is to succeed in and graduate from veterinary school. The long-term goal is to find a particular area of veterinary medicine that I would like to focus on and make a career out of whatever that may be.

What are you doing as an applicant/pre-vet to prepare for veterinary school?
As an early admission student at KSU, I have had the opportunity to explore the veterinary field without worrying about résumé building and the normal application process. To mentally prepare for vet school, I have found extracurricular activities to relieve stress and develop a social network. Additionally, I joined a lab through the vet school that studies mosquito-borne diseases as they relate to animal health.

What extracurricular activities are you involved in currently?
I am very involved in the music scene at my university. Throughout undergrad, I have played with more than eight instrumental ensembles both through the school and across the country. Academically, I have served as a student officer for the microbiology club and worked to provide fellow students with valuable academic opportunities.

How old were you when you first became interested in being a veterinarian?
It wasn't until my junior year of high school that I developed a serious interest in pursuing veterinary medicine. It was at this time that I began regularly volunteering at the local animal shelter.

Please describe your various experiences in preparation for applying to veterinary school.
In preparation for veterinary school, I have shadowed and been employed by large and small animal veterinarians. I have also volunteered for several animal shelters around Kansas and Missouri. More recently, I have spent about 15 hours a week in my laboratory, gaining knowledge on emerging infectious diseases in the veterinary field. As a student in microbiology, I have also taken electives in animal science to develop an adequate background for vet school courses.

What characteristics are you looking for in a veterinary school?
In the US, every accredited veterinary school offers quality education and opportunities to succeed in the field. As an undergraduate student who will likely obtain an advanced degree, a school that provides a broad and encompassing education is one I am most interested in attending. Realistically, the cost of tuition and living expenses is one of the most important aspects of veterinary school for young applicants such as myself.

What advice do you have for other pre-veterinary students?
Don't worry so much about focusing on one aspect of veterinary medicine to pursue. One question we always get as pre-vet students is "small animal or large animal?" In reality, there are so many more things you can do with a DVM degree. Gain experience in several different fields, try undergraduate research, and spend more time doing things you enjoy.

UNIVERSITY OF TENNESSEE

Email Address: dshepherd@utk.edu
Website: http://www.vet.utk.edu

SCHOOL DESCRIPTION

The University of Tennessee's College of Veterinary Medicine is located in Knoxville, a city of 185,000 situated in the Appalachian foothills of east central Tennessee. Only 45 minutes from the Great Smoky Mountains National Park and 3 hours from both Nashville and Atlanta, Knoxville offers many recreational and cultural opportunities, including a symphony orchestra, an opera company, and several fine theaters. The climate in Knoxville is moderate with distinct seasons.

> The Knoxville campus of the University of Tennessee has about 21,300 undergraduate and 6,200 graduate students.

The 550-acre Knoxville campus of the University of Tennessee has about 21,300 undergraduate and 6,200 graduate students. The modern Clyde M. York Veterinary Medicine Building, housing the teaching and research facilities, the Veterinary Medical Center, including the W.W. Armistead Veterinary Teaching Hospital, and Agriculture-Veterinary Medicine Library, faces the Tennessee River on the university's Agricultural Campus.

The curriculum of the College of Veterinary Medicine is a 9-semester, 4-year program. Development of a strong basic science education is emphasized in the first year. The second and third years emphasize the study of diseases, their causes, diagnosis, treatment, and prevention. Innovative features of the first two-and-a-half years of the curriculum include 5 weeks of student-centered small-group applied-learning exercises in semesters 1-5; 3 weeks of dedicated clinical experiences in the Veterinary Medical Center in semesters 3-5; and elective course opportunities in semesters 2-9 that allow students to focus on specific educational/career goals. In the clinical year (final 4 semesters), students participate exclusively in 68 weeks of clinical training (28 weeks of core rotations and 24-30 weeks of elective rotations) in the Veterinary Medical Center and in required off-campus externships. The college has unique programs in zoo, avian, and exotic animal medicine and surgery, cancer diagnosis and therapy, minimally invasive surgery (laser lithotripsy, endoscopy, otoscopy), and rehabilitation/physical therapy.

APPLICATION INFORMATION

For specific application information (availability, deadlines, fees, and VMCAS participation), please refer to the contact information listed above. We admit approximately 85 applicants each year. Priority is given to Tennessee residents (60 of the 85 seats are for Tennessee residents). Twenty-five highly qualified non-residents are admitted each year.

Residency implications: Tennessee has no contractual agreements for residency waivers. Tennessee accepts applications from United States citizens and permanent residents of the United States. Applications from international students completing the recognized prerequisites will be considered for 2018. TOEFL score and international student requirements can be found at http://international.utk.edu.

SUMMARY OF ADMISSION PROCEDURES

Timetable

VMCAS application deadline: Monday, September 17, 2018 at 12 Midnight Eastern Time

PREREQUISITES FOR ADMISSION

General inorganic chemistry (with laboratory)	8
Organic chemistry (with laboratory)	8
General biology/zoology (with laboratory)	8
Cellular/Molecular biology*	3
Genetics	3
Biochemistry (exclusive of laboratory)†	4
Physics (with laboratory)	8
English composition	6
Social sciences/humanities	18

* It is expected that this requirement will be fulfilled by a course in cellular or molecular biology. An upper-division cell or molecular biology course is preferred.

† This should be a complete upper-division course in general cellular and comparative biochemistry. Half of a 2-semester sequence will not satisfy this requirement. Applicants are strongly encouraged to complete additional biological and physical science courses, especially comparative anatomy, mammalian physiology, microbiology with laboratory, and statistics.

GRE scores must be received no later than September 17, 2018

Date interviews are held: TBD in October 2018 and January 2019

Date acceptances mailed: the week of February 18, 2019

Applicant's response date: April 15, 2019

School begins: mid-August 2019

Deposit (to hold place in class): none required.

Deferments: are considered on a case-by-case basis.

EVALUATION CRITERIA

The admission procedure consists of a 3-phased review process (i.e., academic review, packet review, and interview). Each section weighted equally in the final applicant score. The initial academic review determines which applicants will move forward to a packet review. The combined academic review and packet review determines selection of the applicant interview pool.

Initial academic file review includes:
Academic performance and grade point average
GRE Test scores
Prerequisite completion
VMCAS and Supplemental Application information
VMCAS Disadvantaged/Hardship statement (optional)

Holistic packet review:
Rigor of educational program and potential for success
Personal Statement

References (3-5 required – 3 veterinarian letters preferred)
Evidence of logical preparation for this career
Veterinary and Animal Experience
Extracurricular activities/community service
Leadership and diversity
Disadvantaged/Hardship factors
TN: Essay or Personal Statement

Interview:
TN: Personal Statement
Animal/veterinary experience
Communication skills
Motivation
Understanding of the profession
Personal interests and qualities
Professionalism

ENTRANCE REQUIREMENTS

Required undergraduate GPA: for nonresident applicants, the minimum acceptable cumulative GPA is 3.20 on a 4.00 scale. At time of acceptance, the mean GPA of the class entering in fall of 2017 was 3.62.

AP credit policy: must appear on official college transcripts and be equivalent to the appropriate college-level coursework.

Course completion deadline: prerequisite courses must be completed with a grade of C or better by the end of the spring term prior to entry.

Is a Bachelor's Degree Required? no

Is this an International School? no

ESTIMATED TUITION

Estimated Tuition Resident: $28,734

Estimated Tuition Contract: $0

Estimated Tuition Non-Resident: $56,540

AVAILABLE SEATS

Resident: 60

Contract: 0

Non-Resident: 25

TEST REQUIREMENTS

Standardized examinations: Graduate Record Exam (GRE), General Test (Verbal, Quantitative, and Analytical) is required, and scores must be received by September 17, 2018. (To assure scores are reported by the application deadline, applicants should consider exam dates prior to August 15, 2018.)

English Language Requirement: Applicants whose native language is not English are required to take and pass the Test of English as a Foreign Language (TOEFL) or the International English Language Testing System (IELTS). Passing marks are 550, 213, 80, and 6.5 for paper-based, computer-based, internet-based (iBT) TOEFL, and IELTS respectively. Official scores must be received directly from the appropriate testing service. TOEFL scores must be received by January 25, 2019.

The University of Tennessee's score reporting code for TOEFL is 1843. The score must not be older than two years from the requested date of entry. Applicants who have received a degree from an accredited US institution in the past two years are exempt from the TOEFL or IELTS requirement.

TOEFL information may be obtained from the official TOEFL website.

IELTS information may be obtained from the official IELTS website.

VMCAS Participation: full

Accepts International Students? yes

ADDITIONAL INFORMATION

Additional requirements and considerations
 Animal/veterinary work experience
 3 letters of recommendation are required but no more than 5 letters will be accepted. Two should be from veterinarians.
 Extracurricular and/community service activities
 Leadership skills
 Autobiographical essay (personal statement)
 A Supplemental Application is required and an optional Disadvantages Declaration and can be found at: http://www.vet.utk.edu/admissions/supplemental

Dual Degree Program
The College, in partnership with the College of Education, Health and Human Sciences, offers an option for veterinary students (and graduate veterinarians) to earn the MPH degree with a concentration in Veterinary Public Health.

Contact the College of Veterinary Medicine, Dr. Marcy Souza at msouza@utk.edu for additional information.

Dual DVM/PhD Program
The College, in partnership with the Graduate School, offers a dual DVM/PhD program option to students interested in a research career. Students are eligible to take a limited number of courses to count toward a PhD degree in Comparative and Experimental Medicine. Entry to the program requires a separate application to the graduate school. For more information visit http://www.vet.utk.edu/graduate/index.php

*Please see our website for complete information at: https://vetmed.tennessee.edu/admissions/Pages/admissions-process.aspx

TEXAS A&M UNIVERSITY

Email Address: studentadmissions@cvm.tamu.edu
Website: vetmed.tamu.edu

SCHOOL DESCRIPTION

The university is located adjacent to the cities of Bryan and College Station. The two cities have a combined population of approximately 200,000. The student population at Texas A&M is more than 58,000. The College of Veterinary Medicine is one of the 10 original veterinary teaching institutions that existed in the United States prior to World War II.

The College provides an integrated professional curriculum that prepares graduates with a firm foundation in the basic sciences, a broad comparative medicine knowledge base, and the clinical and personal skills to be leaders in the many career fields of veterinary medicine. Professional students are given the opportunity to gain additional education and training in their personal career paths.

> The College of Veterinary Medicine is one of the 10 original teaching institutions that existed in the US prior to World War II.

Becoming a veterinarian requires much dedication and diligent study. The veterinary medical student is required to meet a high level of performance. The demands on students' time and effort are considerable, but the rewards and career satisfaction are personal achievements that make significant contributions to our society.

APPLICATION INFORMATION

For specific application information (availability, deadlines and fees), please refer to the contact information listed above.

Residency implications: Texas has no contractual agreements with other states. Applicants from other states who have outstanding credentials will be considered. Texas seats 132 residents and up to 10 non-resident applicants per year. In the event that not all 10 non-resident positions are filled, these positions will then be filled with Texas alternates. Successful non-resident candidates who are awarded competitive university-based scholarships may attend at the resident tuition rate.

SUMMARY OF ADMISSION PROCEDURES

Timetable

Application deadline: October 1 (5 p.m. CST)

Date interviews are held: January

Date acceptances mailed: mid-March

School begins: late August

Deposit (to hold place in class): none required

Deferments: requests for deferments will be considered on a case-by-case basis

EVALUATION CRITERIA

Academic performance

Test scores

Interview

Personal statement

Evaluations (3 evaluations are required. 1 evaluation must be from a veterinarian with whom you have worked with. No letters of support/recommendation are needed)

PREREQUISITES FOR ADMISSION

Course Description	Number of Hours/Credits	Necessity
General Biology with lab	4	Required
General Microbiology with lab	4	Required
Genetics	3	Required
Animal Nutrition or Feeds & Feeding	3	Required
Inorganic Chemistry I & II with lab	8	Required
Organic Chemistry I & II with lab	8	Required
Biochemistry (lecture hours only)	3	Required
Statistics (upper level)	3	Required
Physics I & II with lab	8	Required
English	6	Required
Public Speaking	3	Required

Semester course load and post-academic challenge

Leadership and experience

ENTRANCE REQUIREMENTS

Required undergraduate GPA: the minimum overall GPA required is 2.90 on a 4.00 scale and 3.10 for the last 45 GPA and 2.90 Science GPA. The mean of the most recent entering class was 3.68.

AP credit policy: AP credit is accepted as fulfilling selected prerequisites; credit must be reflected on the official undergraduate transcript.

Is a Bachelor's Degree Required? no

Is this an International School? no

ESTIMATED TUITION

Estimated Tuition Resident: $22,912

Estimated Tuition Contract: $0

Estimated Tuition Non-Resident: $34,600

AVAILABLE SEATS

Resident: 132

Contract: 0

Non-Resident: 10

TEST REQUIREMENTS

Standardized examinations: Graduate Record Examination (GRE), general test, is required. Beginning August 1, 2011, the College of Veterinary Medicine will require the new version of the GRE examination. Deadline for taking the GRE will be September 30. Scores over 5 years old will not be accepted.

VMCAS Participation: non-VMCAS

Accepts International Students? no

ADDITIONAL INFORMATION

Application Deadline: 10/01/2018 (5 p.m. CST)

TUFTS UNIVERSITY

Email Address: vetadmissions@tufts.edu
Website: vet.tufts.edu

Cummings School
of Veterinary Medicine

SCHOOL DESCRIPTION

Cummings School of Veterinary Medicine at Tufts University is committed to advancing One Health initiatives that enhance the health and well-being of animals, humans and the environment. Cummings School is well-positioned to apply One Health philosophies, leveraging the collective expertise of Tufts University's constellation of health science schools, including veterinary, medical, dental, and nutrition. The University's leadership in both clinical and research settings reaches across disciplines, into the classroom, and out into the world.

> Tufts' leadership in clinical and research settings reaches across disciplines, into the classroom, and into the world.

Our faculty advance science, improve patient care and, most importantly, inspire our students to approach their profession with open minds and a desire to make a difference. The relatively small student body ensures close professional relationships and networking opportunities. An array of curricular options, including electives and dual degree programs, allows each student to find and nurture his or her evolving niche within the profession.

Veterinary students play an integral role in the seven hospitals and clinics that comprise Cummings Veterinary Medical Center at Tufts. From their first year onward, students gain valuable expertise and enjoy a rich clinical learning environment at the:

- Foster Hospital for Small Animals, offering one of the largest small animal caseloads in the country, especially in the area of emergency and critical care where we are designated by the American College of Veterinary Emergency and Critical Care as a national Veterinary Trauma Center.
- Lerner Spay and Neuter Clinic, where students hone their surgical skills.
- Hospital for Large Animals, providing active involvement in the diagnosis, treatment and prevention of disease in horses, especially equine athletes and sport horses, camelids and small ruminants.
- Wildlife Clinic, engaging students in the hands-on practice of wildlife medicine as well as the larger ethical and conservation issues that impact wildlife, people, and the environment.
- Tufts at Tech Community Veterinary Clinic, an innovative, low-cost clinic located within a public technical high school, where students provide primary care to underserved communities in the area.
- Tufts Ambulatory Service, the largest food animal practice in southern New England, addressing health and production needs of cattle, small ruminants and horses. The School's farm, just steps away from the classroom, offers additional hands-on experience in agriculture and food supply veterinary medicine.
- Tufts Veterinary Emergency Treatment and Specialties (Tufts VETS), providing students the opportunity to work in an after-hours urgent care and specialty setting that closely aligns with a private practice business model.

PREREQUISITES FOR ADMISSION

Course Description	Number of Hours/Credits	Necessity
Biology with laboratory	8	Required
Chemistry with laboratory	8	Required
Organic Chemistry with laboratory	8	Required
Biochemistry	3	Required
Physics	6	Required
Genetics*	3	Required
Mathematics/Statistics	6	Required
English/Speech	6	Required
Humanities and Fine Arts	6	Required
Social and Behavioral Sciences	6	Required

* unless included in biology

Students engage in a myriad of opportunities, including basic, translational and clinical research, shelter medicine, comparative oncology, wildlife and conservation medicine, the study of human-animal interactions, regenerative medicine, and more. A major international grant, Emerging Pandemic Threats One Health Workforce, and the International Veterinary Medicine certificate program, along with other ongoing projects, allow students to contribute to global One Health. These opportunities create a campus without boundaries, offer unique learning experiences, and ultimately lead our graduates to exciting and fulfilling careers.

Located just 30 miles west of the city of Boston, students take advantage of the area's internationally renowned teaching hospitals and biomedical research centers, as well as join in the vibrant atmosphere of more than 300,000 college students living, learning, and growing together.

We invite you to explore our website and visit our campus to learn more about Cummings School of Veterinary Medicine at Tufts University: vet.tufts.edu.

APPLICATION INFORMATION

For specific application information (availability, deadlines, fees, and VMCAS participation), please refer to the contact information listed above.

Residency implications: Massachusetts residents make up about one-third of each class.

SUMMARY OF ADMISSION PROCEDURES

Timetable

VMCAS Application Deadline: Monday, September 17, 2018 at 12 Midnight Eastern Time

Date interviews are held: December, January, February

Date acceptances mailed: March

School begins: late August

Deposit (to hold place in class): $500.00

Deferments: requests for deferment are handled on a case-by-case basis.

EVALUATION CRITERIA

Tufts' admission procedure consists of a review of the application and an interview of selected applicants.

ENTRANCE REQUIREMENTS

Required undergraduate GPA: no minimum GPA required. The mean GPA for the Class of 2021 was 3.70.

AP credit policy: must appear on official college transcripts and be equivalent to the appropriate college-level coursework.

Is a Bachelor's Degree Required? no

Is this an International School? no

ESTIMATED TUITION

Estimated Tuition Resident: $50,500

Estimated Tuition Contract: N/A

Estimated Tuition Non-Resident: $55,600

AVAILABLE SEATS

Resident: 30

Contract: 0

Non-Resident: 68

TEST REQUIREMENTS

Standardized examinations: Graduate Record Examinations (GRE), general test, is required. The most recent acceptable test date for applicants to the Class of 2022 is September 17, 2018. Scores are valid for five years. The mean GRE scores for the Class of 2021 were: Verbal 160, Quantitative 158, and Analytical Writing 4.5.

VMCAS Participation: full

Accepts International Students? yes

ADDITIONAL INFORMATION

Application Deadline: 9/17/2018

TUSKEGEE UNIVERSITY

TUSKEGEE
UNIVERSITY

SCHOOL DESCRIPTION

Tuskegee University College of Veterinary Medicine is located in Tuskegee, Alabama, a city of about 13,000. Tuskegee is 40 miles east of the state of Alabama, Capitol City, Montgomery, and twenty miles west of the city of Auburn. It is also within easy driving distance to the cities of Birmingham, Alabama and Atlanta, Georgia. Summers are hot with moderate to mild humidity, and winters are moderate. Its recreational facilities, lakes, and parks can be enjoyed year-round.

Since it was founded by Booker T. Washington in 1881, Tuskegee University (HBCU) has become one of our nation's most outstanding institutions of higher learning. While it focuses on helping to develop human resources primarily within the African-American community, it is open to all.

Tuskegee's mission has always been to provide service to people in addition to education. The University stresses the need to educate the whole person, that is, the hand and the heart as well as the mind. Tuskegee enrolls more than 3,000 students and employs approximately 900 faculty and support personnel. Physical facilities include more than 5,000 acres of forestry and a campus consisting of more than 100 major buildings and structures. Total land, forestry, and facilities are valued in excess of $500 million. The campus has also been declared a historical site by the United States Department of the Interior.

> The University stresses the need to educate the whole person, that is, the hand and the heart as well as the mind.

Historically, Tuskegee University College of Veterinary Medicine (TUCVM) was established in 1945 for the training of African-Americans during a time when few had the opportunity to study veterinary medicine because of segregation and other racial impediments.

The Tuskegee University College of Veterinary Medicine (TUCVM) was established in 1945 and is the only veterinary medical professional program located on the campus of a Historically Black College or University (HBCU) in the United States. The TUCVM has educated over 70 percent of the Nation's African American veterinarians, and is recognized as the most diverse of all 30 Schools/Colleges of Veterinary Medicine in the U.S. The primary mission of the TUCVM is to provide an environment that nurtures and promotes a spirit of active, independent and self-directed learning, teaching, research and service in veterinary medicine and related disciplines.

Also, TUCVM's graduates have excelled in private clinical practice, public practice such the government, military, and in corporations such as the pharmaceutical industry. They hold key leadership positions in the government, military, academia, and in the international arena.

APPLICATION INFORMATION

Supplemental application fee: TUCVM requires a $100.00 supplemental fee. Send supplemental application fee directly to: Office of Veterinary Admissions and Recruitment, Tuskegee University College of Veterinary Medicine, 1200 West Montgomery Rd, Tuskegee Institute, Al 36088.

For specific application information (availability, deadlines, fees, and VMCAS), please refer to

PREREQUISITES FOR ADMISSION

Courses and Requirements in Semester Hours

I. English or Written Composition	6
II. Mathematics	6
III. Social Sciences / Humanities	6
IV. Liberal Arts	6
	24
V. Biological & Physical Sciences	
Advance Biology (300 Level or Above)**	9
Biochemistry w/Lab	4
Advance Biology Electives	8
Chemistry w/Lab	4
Organic Chemistry w/Lab	4
Physics w/Lab	8
	37
VI. Medical Terminology	1
Physical Education	2
VII. Animal Science	
Introduction to Animal Science	3
Animal Nutrition	3
	6
Total Semester Hours	**70**

** Advanced biology courses, e.g., anatomy, physiology, ecology, immunology, zoology, microbiology, genetics, toxicology, and histology

All required science courses (Advance biology, biochemistry, chemistry, physics) must have been completed within six (6) calendar years of the time of admission.

the contact information listed above, or visit the online application process at: http://aavmc.org/Students -Applicants-and-Advisors/Veterinary-Medical-College -Application-Service.aspx.

Residency implications: applications are accepted with special consideration given to Alabama residents and those who have residency in the following contract states, Kentucky, and South Carolina.

Number of resident seats and non-resident seats: none - TUCVM maintains "open access" and selection for seats.

International applications will be considered for admissions into TUCVM.

PREREQUISITES FOR ADMISSION

The Tuskegee University College of Veterinary Medicine's professional curriculum is a rigorous four-year program. Therefore applicant's final grade for each required course must be a "C" or better. Students are required to take the General Aptitude portion of the Graduate Record Examination (GRE). Applicants must submit an analytical writing score along with the GRE. Additionally, there is a mandatory interview with the TUCVM Admissions Committee before acceptance into the school is granted.

GPA: the minimum cumulative and science GPA requirement is 3.0 on a 4.00 scale.

Course completion deadline: Applicants must complete all prerequisites by the end of the spring semester preceding matriculation. All final transcripts are required to be submitted to TUCVM, not VMCAS by June 1.

Tuskegee requires a minimum of 200 clinical contact hours with a licensed veterinarian.

Standardized examinations of the application year: Graduate Record Examination (GRE) of which must be taken within three years of application, is required. Must be completed by September 1. Request GRE Test Scores results by October 1.

SUMMARY OF ADMISSION PROCEDURE

Timetable

VMCAS application deadline: September 17 at 12 Midnight Eastern Time

Date interviews are held: January-February

Date offers of acceptances mailed: March

School begins: mid-August

Deferments: one-year deferments are considered on a case-by-case basis.

EVALUATION CRITERIA

The following items are taken into consideration: academic record, academic trends, letters of recommendation, work experience, and test scores.

	% weight
Grades	68
Test scores	8
Animal/veterinary experience	6
Interview	15
References	
Science Professors	2
Veterinarian	1
Essay (Handwritten, see application)	

Number of available seats: Approximately 60-65

EXPENSES FOR THE 2018–2019 ACADEMIC YEAR

Tuition and fees

Tuition: $20,585 per semester

Technology fee: $500.00

I.D. fee: $30.00

Supplemental application fee: $100.00

If admitted, additional fees and expenses are required.

DUAL-DEGREE PROGRAMS

Combined DVM–Graduate Degree Programs are available: PhD in Integrative Biosciences, PhD Interdisciplinary Pathobiology, Master of Science Veterinary Science, Master of Public Health and Master of Science in Public Health.

FIRST-YEAR PROFILE: SHAWN KOZLOV

Current School Name
Virginia-Maryland College of Veterinary Medicine

Why do you want to be a veterinarian?
I was initially drawn to the veterinary profession with an interest in biological science and a compassion for animals. This opened my eyes to a profession with a wide-ranging impact on animal lives, human lives, and the environment. There is no shortage of opportunities to make a difference in the world for veterinarians either in small animal practices, biomedical research, or public health. The more I learned about this robust world, the greater my desire became to continue my career in the veterinary field by pursing a degree in veterinary medicine.

What are your short-term and long-term goals?
My short-term goals include being successful and involved in the veterinary program at the Virginia Maryland College of Veterinary Medicine. I am President of the Class of 2021 and want to both succeed and help my classmates succeed in becoming well-qualified, competent members of the field I have come to love. I hope to find a surgery residency where I can put my many years of lab animal surgery experience to good use and learn to be a leader in the animal surgery field.

Long-term, I look forward to contributing to the veterinary field through mentoring, presenting, and maybe one day returning to teach the next generation of veterinary students. I would like to someday be as influential and encouraging to future veterinary students as so many great veterinarians have been to me. I am not sure where my career in veterinary medicine will take me, but I know that one of the great things about being a veterinarian is that you have many diverse and amazing opportunities.

What did you do as an applicant to prepare for applying to veterinary school?
The first piece of advice I would offer to potential applicants is to understand the challenges facing the veterinary field after graduation. It is important to understand the cost of veterinary school both monetarily and emotionally. If the opportunities available as a veterinarian are still appealing—and they certainly are for me—then be prepared for a challenge. The second piece of advice I would give an applicant is to not give up easily. I did not get into a veterinary school my first attempt, and I am very happy I spoke with the admission offices at the schools I was rejected from and tried again.

What advice would you give to applicants or those considering applying to veterinary school?
Be sure—really sure—that it's what you want. Work with, shadow, and talk to vets who are living the career you want; ask them about the difficult, unpleasant, challenging parts of their work. Vet school is just too large an investment of money, time, opportunity-cost, and stress to take on, with anything less than complete confidence in your decision.

What helped make the transition to veterinary school easier for you?
The transition to veterinary school was startling for me at first. I am a nontraditional student who had been working full time for many years. I decided to get involved and make connections with other students and faculty as quickly as possible. This allowed me to feel more like I belonged and less like an imposter. I believe this is good advice for both nontraditional and traditional students. I felt like I was immediately a part of a team working toward my success.

What is your advice on student debt?
Understand it! Understand how loans work, how the repayment plans work, and what veterinarians working in your field of interest typically make. The more you know and understand about the loan and repayment process, the better prepared you can be to make decisions throughout the application and education process. This can help relieve any loan stress you might feel throughout school and when you graduate.

What are you most excited about learning in veterinary school?
As cliché as it might sound, I am excited to learn everything. I have been lucky enough to work in the veterinary field for many years, and I have a good understanding of a lot of concepts. I am excited to learn the details that fill in the blanks and connect concepts of which I had previously only scratched the surface. After my first semester of classes, I have already expanded so much, and I can't wait to expand on everything else.

VIRGINIA-MARYLAND
COLLEGE OF VETERINARY MEDICINE

Email Address: dvmadmit@vt.edu
Website: www.becomeavet.vetmed.vt.edu

SCHOOL DESCRIPTION

The Virginia-Maryland College of Veterinary Medicine is situated on the campus of Virginia Tech in Blacksburg, Virginia. Blacksburg is located in southwest Virginia between the Blue Ridge and Allegheny Mountains and is a distinct community with a population of about 40,000. Its residents enjoy a wide range of educational, social, recreational, and cultural opportunities. In addition to the main campus in Blacksburg, there are two other campuses, the Equine Medical Center, located in Leesburg, Virginia, and the Gudelsky Center, which is located on the campus of the University of Maryland, College Park.

> Comprehensive four-year curriculum enables students to integrate knowledge, skills, and professional attributes.

Our comprehensive four-year curriculum enables students to integrate their knowledge, skills, and professional attributes within diverse learning environments, all while focusing on the major areas of veterinary medicine. Students will gain proficiency while learning in the large classroom, small group integrative sessions, the clinical skills center, and laboratories. After two years of preclinical coursework, students will begin their first clinical experience. The clinical teaching time spans two summer semesters, after which students will immerse themselves in higher level coursework within one of five emphasis areas. At the end of this second teaching time, students will complete their extensive veterinary training within the clinical setting.

APPLICATION INFORMATION

For specific application information (availability, deadlines, fees, and VMCAS participation), please refer to our website at: http://www.becomeavet.vetmed.vt.edu

Residency implications: 50 positions are reserved for Virginia residents, and 30 positions for Maryland residents. Up to 40 additional positions may be filled by nonresidents, 6 of those reserved for WV residents.

SUMMARY OF ADMISSION PROCEDURES

Timetable

Supplemental application deadline: September 17, 2018 (The supplemental application can be accessed at: www.becomeavet.vetmed.vt.edu/howto/steps_to_apply, and will open on May 15, 2018.)

Date interviews are held: January 18 and 19, 2019

Date acceptances mailed: February 14, 2019

School begins: August 19, 2019

Deposit (to hold place in class): $400 for residents and non-residents

Deferments: case-by-case basis if a candidate has extenuating circumstances beyond his or her control

EVALUATION CRITERIA

The admission procedure is comprised of an initial screening of applicants, review of the application portfolios, and interviews of selected applicants.

PREREQUISITES FOR ADMISSION

Course Description	Number of Hours/Credits	Necessity
General Biology	8	Required
Organic Chemistry	6	Required
General or Introductory Physics	8	Required
Biochemistry	3	Required
Humanities/Social Sciences	6	Required
Math: algebra, geometry, trigonometry, calculus, or statistics	6	Required
English (3 semester hours must be English composition or a writing-intensive designated course)	6	Required

Pre-Interview Evaluation

60%: Academics: cumulative GPA, required science GPA, last 45 semester hour GPA

40%: Non-Academics: related animal experience, veterinary experience; research, industrial, and biomedical experiences; references; and overall application portfolio review

Interviews

Top candidates ranked on the above criteria will be invited to participate in the Multi Mini Interview process. Admissions offers will be based on interview results.

ENTRANCE REQUIREMENTS

Students must earn a "C-" or better in all required courses.

Science courses taken 7 or more years ago may be repeated or substituted with higher-level courses with the written consent of the admissions committee.

Advanced placement credit for 1 semester of English will be accepted if the additional required hours are composition or technical writing and are taken at a college or university.

Advanced placement credit or credit by examination for preveterinary course requirements will be accepted. Those credits must appear on the applicant's college transcript. Advanced placement credits will not be calculated in grade point averages and no grade assigned. No course substitutions will be allowed for AP credit or credit by examination.

Course completion deadline: required courses must be completed by the end of the spring term of the year in which matriculation occurs.

Standardized examinations: GRE not required.

Letters of recommendation: Letters of recommendations are not required. However, letters of recommendation may be submitted electronically through VMCAS and will be reviewed with the rest of the application.

ADDITIONAL REQUIREMENTS AND CONSIDERATIONS

Maturity and a broad cultural perspective

Evidence of potential, and appreciation of the career opportunities for veterinarians, as indicated by:
1. Clinical veterinary experience (private practice)
2. Animal experience in addition to time spent working with a veterinarian
3. Biomedical/research experience (such as working with veterinarians or other biomedically trained individuals in health care, government, research laboratories, industrial, or corporate settings.)
4. Extramural activities, achievements, honors
5. Communication skills

Is a Bachelor's Degree Required? no

Is this an International School? no

ESTIMATED TUITION

Estimated Tuition Resident: $24,197

Estimated Tuition Contract: $51,966 per year*

Estimated Tuition Non-Resident: $51,966 per year

*West Virginia Higher Education Council provides scholarship money for a portion of tuition.

AVAILABLE SEATS

Virginia Residents: 50

Maryland Residents: 30

West Virginia Contract Seats: 6

Non-Residents: 34

VMCAS Participation: full

Accepts International Students? yes

ADDITIONAL INFORMATION

Application Deadline: 9/17/2018

WASHINGTON STATE UNIVERSITY

Email Address: admissions@vetmed.wsu.edu
Website: www.dvm.vetmed.wsu.edu

WASHINGTON STATE
UNIVERSITY

SCHOOL DESCRIPTION

The Washington-Idaho-Montana-Utah (WIMU) Regional Program in Veterinary Medicine is a partnership between the Washington State University College of Veterinary Medicine, University of Idaho Department of Animal and Veterinary Science, Montana State University, and Utah State University School of Veterinary Medicine. Our program accepts students from all of our contract states and seats are available for non-residents on both the WSU and USU campuses. The WSU College of Veterinary Medicine is also a partner with the Western Interstate Commission of Higher Education (WICHE) program and welcomes WICHE-sponsored students from Arizona, Hawaii, Montana, Nevada, New Mexico, North Dakota, and Wyoming.

> The Washington-Idaho-Montana-Utah (WIMU) Regional Program in Veterinary Medicine is a partnership.

Washington State University

Washington State University is in Pullman, a town in southeastern Washington. Located in the Palouse region of the Inland Northwest, Pullman offers the benefits of small-town living with the cultural richness of bigger city life. The 60,000 people who live in the communities of Pullman and neighboring town, Moscow, Idaho, enjoy a lifestyle that combines a beautiful country setting with the benefits of two major universities (University of Idaho is just a few miles away). WSU is also a member of the PAC-12 athletic conference, offering exciting sporting events throughout the year. With a true four-season climate, beautiful rivers, nearby mountains and scenic mountain lakes, it's easy to take advantage of a variety of excellent recreational activities including hiking, mountain biking, skiing, snowboarding, fishing, camping and whitewater rafting.

The WSU College of Veterinary Medicine was founded in 1899 and is one of the longest established colleges of veterinary medicine in the country. Several major buildings house the Departments of Veterinary Clinical Sciences, Integrative Physiology and Neuroscience, Veterinary Microbiology and Pathology, and the School of Molecular Biosciences. The college also includes the Veterinary Teaching Hospital, the Washington Animal Disease Diagnostic Laboratory and the Paul G. Allen School for Global Animal Health.

Hands-on experience at WSU begins on day one with caseloads that provide extensive experience in all areas of interest including small animal, food animal, equine, and exotics. Because WSU clinicians have a wide range of specialty areas, the Veterinary Teaching Hospital sees a large and diverse caseload. Students are encouraged to spend time in the Veterinary Teaching Hospital throughout all four years of study. The DVM program also allows for students to take advantage of numerous off-campus clinical opportunities in all areas of veterinary medicine. There are interactive case opportunities at our satellite locations in Spokane, Washington, and southern Idaho, our primary care programs in partnership with the Seattle Humane Society and Idaho Humane Society, and our affiliate preceptor clinics scattered throughout the Northwest.

The WSU College of Veterinary Medicine is also a leader of innovative educational programs. Before students even take their first veterinary class, they begin their education with an on-site and off-site retreat designed to promote collaboration and team building. By

PREREQUISITES FOR ADMISSION	
Course requirements and semester hours	
Biology (with lab)	8
Inorganic chemistry (with lab)	8
Organic chemistry (with lab)	4
Physics (with lab)	4
Math (algebra or higher)	3
Genetics	3-4
Biochemistry	3
Statistical methods	3
Arts/Humanities/Social Sciences/History*	21
English composition/Communication*	6
TOTAL	**64**

*General education requirements will be waived if a student has a bachelor's degree.

the time students enter their second year, in addition to the veterinary curriculum, they have already studied ethics, service, and leadership in veterinary medicine. In their second and third years, students take classes to learn skills in clinical communication, diagnostic reasoning, and may elect to take courses on how to manage a veterinary practice as a part of the Veterinary Business Management Association Certificate Program. Students at WSU have multiple opportunities to engage in dynamic research programs throughout all four years. Opportunities include the Research Scholars Program, Summer Research Program, Research Elective/Supplemental Core Courses, Northwest Bovine Veterinary Experience Program, and combined DVM/graduate studies.

Utah State University
Utah State University is nationally and internationally recognized for its research in animal and biomedical sciences. USU's School of Veterinary Medicine offers an academically outstanding path to pursue a professional degree in veterinary medicine. Classes are taught by faculty from the Department of Animal, Dairy, and Veterinary Sciences and are held in state-of-the-art teaching facilities on the Logan, Utah campus. With dedicated faculty and up to 30 students per class, students will experience a supportive environment for active learning. Students spend their first two years in Logan and then transfer to Pullman for their remaining two years.

Cache Valley is one of Utah's hidden treasures, and Logan, with its population of approximately 50,000 residents, sits at the heart of it. Cache Valley lies 83 miles north of Salt Lake City and is a land of dairy farms, small towns, and friendly people. The majestic mountains provide outstanding all-season outdoor recreation, and there are plenty of historical, musical, and art events, plus numerous dining, lodging, and shopping offerings.

Montana State University
Montana State University is a public university located in Bozeman, Montana. It is the state's land grant university and primary campus in the Montana State University System. MSU is ranked in the top tier of US research institutions by the Carnegie Foundation for the Advancement of Teaching. Montana residents spend their first year in Bozeman and then transfer to Pullman for their remaining three years.

Bozeman is located in the beautiful Gallatin Valley, and is a safe and supportive community offering significant opportunity to combine a fantastic educational experience with the great outdoors. Bozeman has a population close to 42,000 residents, making it the fourth largest city in Montana. The area offers fantastic hiking and backpacking opportunities in the surrounding mountain ranges, and the skiing and fishing is some of the best in the country. Yellowstone National Park is a short drive to the south, offering year round recreational activities.

WIMU and WICHE Program Details

Students applying as Washington residents are competing for up to 55 spots for Washington residents only. Students applying as Idaho residents are competing for up to 11 spots for Idaho residents only. Students accepted from the Washington and Idaho pools complete all four years on the WSU Pullman campus. The joint program between WSU/USU seats up to 20 Utah residents and up to 10 nonresidents to spend their first two years in Logan, Utah. Much of the curriculum is taught by the faculty of USU's Department of Animal, Dairy, and Veterinary Sciences, paralleling the curriculum taught in Pullman. The final two years are completed at the WSU Pullman campus. Students applying as Montana residents are competing for up to 10 spots for Montana residents as a part of the regional cooperative program. Students selected for this joint program spend their first year in Bozeman, Montana, where classes, which parallel those in Pullman, are taught by experienced health science educators. The final three years are completed at the WSU Pullman campus. There are up to 25 spots available for WICHE-sponsored and non-resident students at the WSU Pullman Campus.

Upon satisfactory completion of our program, the Doctor of Veterinary Medicine (DVM) degree is conferred by the Regents of Washington State University. Although the University of Idaho, Montana State University, and Utah State University are partners in the program, all students receive their DVM degrees from Washington State University.

APPLICATION INFORMATION

All applicants, regardless of residency, must complete the VMCAS application and WSU/WIMU Supplemental Application. Applicants must declare their state of residency on the VMCAS and WSU/WIMU Supplemental Application. By identifying yourself as a Washington resident, Idaho resident, Montana resident, Utah resident, a resident of a WICHE state (Arizona, Hawaii, Montana, Nevada, New Mexico, North Dakota, Wyoming), or as a nonresident, your application will be funneled through the appropriate application pool. It is highly recommended that applicants contact the appropriate state authority for information regarding residency requirements as early in the application process as possible.

For the most current application information (details, availability, deadlines, fees, and VMCAS participation), please refer to www.dvm.vetmed.wsu.edu as well as the contact information listed above.

Residency implications: In general, first preference is given to qualified applicants who are residents of Washington, Idaho, Montana, Utah, and qualified applicants sponsored by WICHE contract states. Second preference is given to qualified nonresident applicants.

At the Pullman site there are up to 55 available seats for Washington residents, up to 11 for Idaho residents, and up to 25 for WICHE-sponsored and nonresident students.

At the Logan site there are up to 20 available seats for Utah residents and up to 10 for nonresident students.

At the Montana site there are up to 10 available seats for Montana residents.

SUMMARY OF ADMISSIONS PROCEDURES

Timetable

VMCAS application deadline: Monday, September 17, 2018 at 12 Midnight Eastern Time

WSU/WIMU Supplemental deadline: Monday, September 24, 2018 by 5 PM Pacific Time (The supplemental application can be accessed at: www.dvm.vetmed.wsu.edu)

Interview dates: November-February

Acceptance letters mailed: November-April

School begins: late August

Deposit (to hold place in class): none required

Deferments: considered on a case-by-case basis

EVALUATION CRITERIA

Applicants are selected based upon ability to successfully complete the program and demonstration of the qualities that make a successful veterinarian. Academic criteria include grades, quality and rigor of academic program, and GRE test scores. Non-cognitive factors include animal, veterinary, research, and work experience; honors and awards; community service and extracurricular activities; written essay; and letters of recommendation. Other factors include maturity, integrity, compassion, communication skills, and desire to contribute to society. An interview is required for Washington, Idaho, Montana, and Utah residents, as well as for nonresident applicants. WICHE applicants who are certified as residents of their contract state are ranked for participation in the WICHE program using the same criteria above minus the interview.

2017 ADMISSIONS SUMMARY

	Number of Applicants	Number of New Entrants
Washington	158	46
Idaho	41	11
Montana	34	10
Utah	45	19
WICHE states	143	28
(20 WICHE sponsored)		
Nonresident	1,072	19
Total	**1,493**	**133**

(93 Pullman / 30 Logan / 10 Bozeman)

EXPENSES FOR THE 2017-2018 ACADEMIC YEAR

Tuition and fees - Pullman Site

Resident (WA, ID, and WICHE supported): $25,934

Nonresident: $59,164

Tuition and fees - Bozeman Site

Resident: $23,657

Tuition and fees - Logan Site

Resident: $24,428

Nonresident with scholarship: $49,058

Nonresident without scholarship: $57,658

ENTRANCE REQUIREMENTS

Required undergraduate GPA: No minimum requirement.

AP credit policy: Must meet Washington State University requirements.

Course completion deadline: Prerequisite courses must be completed before time of matriculation.

Standardized examinations: Graduate Record Examination (GRE) General Test is required. Test scores older than 5 years will not be accepted. Test scores are due by September 17, 2018.

ADDITIONAL REQUIREMENTS AND CONSIDERATIONS

Animal/veterinary/research/work experience

Letters of Recommendation. Both an academic and DVM letter are required. A minimum of three letters and a maximum of six letters will be reviewed by the admissions committee.

Extracurricular and community service activities, honors and awards

Personal Statement

WSU/WIMU Supplemental Application

Is a Bachelor's Degree Required? no

Is this an International School? no

TEST REQUIREMENTS

Standardized examinations: Graduate Record Examination (GRE) General Test is required. Test scores older than 5 years will not be accepted. Test scores are due by September 17, 2018.

VMCAS Participation: full

Accepts International Students? yes

ADDITIONAL INFORMATION

VMCAS Application Deadline: 9/17/2018

WSU/WIMU Application Deadline: 9/24/2018

WESTERN UNIVERSITY OF HEALTH SCIENCES

Email Address: admissions@westernu.edu
Website: www.prospective.westernu.edu
/veterinary/requirements-17
Link to Application: prospective.westernu.edu
/veterinary/apply-17

SCHOOL DESCRIPTION

Western University of Health Sciences is an independent, accredited, nonprofit university incorporated in the State of California, dedicated to educating compassionate and competent health professionals who value diversity and a humanistic approach to patient care. The university, located in the San Gabriel Valley of Southern California, about 30 miles east of Los Angeles, grants post baccalaureate professional degrees in nine colleges: the College of Podiatric Medicine, the College of Dental Medicine, the College of Optometry, the Graduate College of Biomedical Sciences, the College of Allied Health Professions, the College of Graduate Nursing, the College of Osteopathic Medicine of the Pacific, the College of Pharmacy, and the College of Veterinary Medicine. The American Veterinary Medical Association Council on Education granted the College of Veterinary Medicine full accreditation status in 2010. Western U's CVM admitted its charter class Fall 2003. The founding principles of the College of Veterinary Medicine include:

> Western University is dedicated to educating compassionate and competent health professionals.

1. Commitment to student-centered, life-long learning. The curriculum is designed to teach students to find and critically evaluate information, to enhance student cooperative learning, and to provide an environment for professional development.

2. Commitment to a Reverence for Life philosophy in teaching veterinary medicine. The College strives to make the educational experience one that enhances moral development of its students and is respectful to all animals and people involved in its programs. Students only practice clinical and surgical skills on live animals when it is medically necessary for that animal.

3. Commitment to excellence of student education through strategic partnerships in the public and private veterinary sectors.

This commitment seeks to maximize the learning experience in veterinary clinical practice and to educate practice-ready veterinarians capable of functioning independently upon graduation. In the 3rd and 4th years of the curriculum students are trained primarily off-campus at state of the art facilities.

APPLICATION INFORMATION

For specific application information (availability, deadlines, fees, and VMCAS participation), please refer to the contact information listed previously.

Residency implications: applicants from all states as well as international applicants will be considered. In-state and out-of-state applicants are given equal consideration.

SUMMARY OF ADMISSION PROCEDURES

Timetable

VMCAS application deadline: Monday, September 17, 2018 at 12 Midnight Eastern Time

Supplemental application deadline: electronically submitted with the prerequisite worksheet RECEIVED on or before Monday, September 17, 2018 at 12 PM PST

PREREQUISITES FOR ADMISSION

Course Description	Number of Hours/Credits	Necessity
Organic Chemistry with Lab	3	Required
Biochemistry or Physiological Chemistry	3	Required
Upper-Division Biological and Life Sciences with Lab	9	Required
Microbiology	3	Required
Upper-Division Physiology (Animal, Human, or Comparative Only)	3	Required
Genetics	3	Required
General or College Physics with Labs	6	Required
Statistics (General, Introductory, or Bio-)	3	Required
English Composition	6	Required
Humanities/Social Sciences	9	Required

Date interviews are held: late fall and early spring

Date acceptances mailed: March

School begins: August

Deposit (to hold place in class): $500

Deferments: request for deferments will be considered on a case-by-case basis and only after deposit is received.

EVALUATION CRITERIA

Academic achievement

Standardized test performance

Animal experience

Letters of reference

Interview

Other supporting material

Entrance Requirements

Required undergraduate GPA: Applicants must have a minimum overall GPA of 2.75 (undergraduate and graduate) at the time of application to be considered for admission. Prerequisite courses must be completed with a grade of C (or its equivalent) or higher. GPA must be maintained through matriculation into the program.

AP credit policy: must appear on official college transcripts and be equivalent to the appropriate college-level coursework. AP test subject and number of credits must also be specified on the transcript.

Is a Bachelor's Degree Required? no

Is this an International School? no

ESTIMATED TUITION (2017-2018)

Estimated Tuition Resident: $52,860

Estimated Tuition Contract: $0

Estimated Tuition Non-Resident: $52,860

AVAILABLE SEATS

Resident: 47

Contract: 0

Non-Resident: 53

TEST REQUIREMENTS

Standardized examinations: Graduate Record Examination (GRE), general test, or Medical College Admissions Test (MCAT) is required. Test scores must be RECEIVED by the VMCAS on or before the VMCAS deadline.

VMCAS Participation: full

Accepts International Students? yes

ADDITIONAL INFORMATION

All courses must be completed at a regionally accredited college or university in the United States. Exceptions will be made on a case-by-case basis.

Coursework completed outside the U.S. (including Canada) must be evaluated by a WesternU approved evaluation service (please visit the requirements page of the website for a listing of approved services).

All required courses must be completed by the end of the spring term of planned matriculation year.

Failure to satisfactorily complete prerequisites with a grade of C or better will result in the loss of a candidate's seat in the class.

One course cannot be used to satisfy more than one prerequisite.

All except two of the science prerequisite courses must be completed by the end of the Fall term immediately prior to the planned year of matriculation at WesternU-CVM.

Application Deadline: 9/17/2018

PRE-VETERINARY PROFILE: BRIANNE GRYSPEERD

Current School Name
Oakland University

What type of veterinary medicine are you interested in pursuing, and why?
I am interested in pursuing small-animal veterinary medicine (like canine, feline, and other small mammals). This specific area interests me because the majority of veterinarians I have shadowed are in this field. I grew up with dogs and cats (no farm animals of my own), and those are the kinds of animals I would like to work with in the future.

What is/was your major during undergraduate school?
Biological sciences.

What are your short-term and long-term goals?
My short-term goals are to finish my first year of college in good academic standing. I am also looking for an internship, job, or summer-long shadowing experience with a veterinarian clinic in 2018. One of my goals includes completing at least 10 hours of community service with an animal shelter.

Some of my long-term goals include graduating from Oakland University and graduating from Oakland's Honors College. In or after 2018, I plan to get involved with some sort of animal-related research on campus. I then plan to apply for veterinary school and hopefully go to Michigan State or another university after my undergraduate degree. After vet school, I would be very interested in working with sled dogs in Alaska or northern Canada for a few years.

What are you doing as an applicant/pre-vet to prepare for veterinary school?
To prepare for veterinary school, I am researching the different school options and taking the required classes. I am also trying to build hours in work experience (a job at McDonald's), veterinary work experience (job shadowing), undergraduate research, and animal-related community service (volunteering at shelters).

What extracurricular activities are you involved in currently?
My extracurricular activities include being an active member in the Honors College Student Association and the Pre-Veterinary Medicine Association at Oakland. I am also a part of the 4-H club, K-9 and Kompany, where I show animals, complete community service, and educate youth.

How old were you when you first became interested in being a veterinarian?
I have wanted to be a veterinarian all my life. Throughout middle and high school, I showed dogs and discovered my passion for animals. I also love science classes (specifically biology), so the educational aspect of veterinary medicine is also very interesting. After job shadowing for two summers during high school, I was certain veterinary medicine was my dream career.

Please describe your various experiences in preparation for applying to veterinary school.
As a freshman in college, I have been learning more about the application process and trying to build hours that may set me apart from other applicants. I plan to demonstrate that I have a strong academic background with grades in my major, and that I am well rounded with my work and service experiences. I have around fifty hours of job shadowing experience with veterinarians from recent years.

What characteristics are you looking for in a veterinary school?
I am looking for a veterinary school close to Michigan. Within the neighboring states would be ideal; however, I am interested in some colleges on the west side of the country.

What advice do you have for other pre-veterinary students?
My advice to other pre-vet students is to focus on other areas of applying to vet school, not just the grades. Good academic standing is great, but the experiences an individual has endured improve how they view the field more than anything else can.

UNIVERSITY OF WISCONSIN

Email Address: oaa@vetmed.wisc.edu
Website: www.vetmed.wisc.edu

WISCONSIN
UNIVERSITY OF WISCONSIN–MADISON

SCHOOL DESCRIPTION

The University of Wisconsin is located in Madison, the state capital, which has a population of about 240,000. Consistently ranked among the nation's "most livable" cities, its hilly terrain, scattered parks, and woodlands saturate the urban setting with a friendly neighborhood atmosphere. Centered on a narrow isthmus among 4 scenic lakes, the city is a recreational paradise. The university sprawls over 900 acres along Lake Mendota and its student population is nearly 45,000. It has rated among the top 10 universities academically since 1910 and is sixth in the country in volume of research activity.

> The University of Wisconsin rated among the top 10 universities academically since 1910.

The School of Veterinary Medicine facility has a modern veterinary medical teaching hospital, modern equipment, and high-quality lab space for teaching and research. The curriculum provides a broad education in veterinary medicine with learning experiences in food animal medicine and other specialty areas. The school pioneered a unique senior rotation in ambulatory service for fourth-year students where they experience the life and work of a veterinarian specializing in large-animal medicine by completing a rotation in one of 24 practices near Madison. The school has an outstanding research program and many faculty members have joint appointments with the College of Agricultural and Life Sciences, the School of Medicine and Public Health, the Wisconsin National Primate Research Center, the McArdle Laboratory for Cancer Research, the National Wildlife Health Laboratory, and the North Central Dairy Forage Center. These outside links provide learning, research, and employment opportunities for students.

APPLICATION INFORMATION

To apply for admission, all applicants must complete three (3) online applications: 1) VMCAS, due September 17, 2018 (12:00 Midnight, EDT); 2) Wisconsin's Required Applicant Data Form, due September 18, 2018 (4:00 p.m., CDT) and located at our website: www.vetmed.wisc.edu/radf; and 3) Wisconsin's Supplemental Application. All applicants will be notified by e-mail in November 2018 to complete our electronic supplemental application and to announce its deadline. Interviews are not required as part of the application process.

For specific application information (availability, deadlines, fees, and VMCAS participation), please refer to our website: https://www.vetmed.wisc.edu.

Residency implications: at least 60 Wisconsin residents will be accepted. Wisconsin has no contractual agreements, but may accept approximately 30 nonresident applicants. Applicants who can claim legal residency or domicile in more than one state should contact the school.

SUMMARY OF ADMISSION PROCEDURES

Timetable

VMCAS application deadline: Monday, September 17, 2018 at 12 Midnight Eastern Time

Interviews: none

Date acceptances mailed: late-February

School begins: late August

PREREQUISITES FOR ADMISSION

Course Description	Number of Hours/Credits	Necessity
Biology or Zoology	4	Required
Genetics or Animal Breeding	3	Required
General Chemistry	8	Required
Organic Chemistry	3	Required
Biochemistry	3	Required
General Physics	6	Required
Statistics	3	Required
English Composition or Journalism	6	Required
Social Science or Humanities	6	Required
Anatomy	3	Recommended
Microbiology	3	Recommended
Physiology	3	Recommended
Cell/Molecular Biology	3	Recommended

Deposit (to hold place in class): none required

Deferments: are considered on an individual basis by the Admissions Committee and may be granted for extenuating circumstances.

EVALUATION CRITERIA

There is a 2-part admission procedure. For the fall 2017 application year, the class was selected based upon the following comparative evaluation:

1. Academic factors, including:
   Undergraduate cumulative GPA
   Required coursework GPA
   Last 30 semester credit GPA
   GRE test scores

2. Non-academic factors, including:
   Animal and veterinary medical experience
   Extracurricular activities and other work experience
   Awards and honors
   Communication skills, maturity and leadership
   Letters of recommendation

ENTRANCE REQUIREMENTS

Required undergraduate GPA: A minimum grade of C (2.0) must be earned in all required courses, including courses completed after application. The mean undergraduate cumulative GPA for the class of 2021 was 3.56 for residents and 3.75 for nonresidents.

AP credit policy: must appear on official college transcripts and be equivalent to the appropriate college-level coursework.

Is a Bachelor's Degree Required? no

Is this an International School? no

ESTIMATED TUITION

Tuition rates are published each year in July; please see our website for details.

2018-2019 Estimated Tuition Resident: $29,626

Estimated Tuition Contract: n/a

2018-2019 Estimated Tuition Non-Resident: $47,770

TEST REQUIREMENTS

Standardized examinations: Graduate Record Examination (GRE), general test, is required. All applicants are required to take or retake the GRE, including the writing assessment. The deadline by which this must be completed is listed on our website. For the most current GRE submission information, please see our website.

A test of English as a foreign language (TOEFL, MELAB, or IELTS scores may be submitted) is required for applicants for whom English is a second language and have not completed an undergraduate degree at an English-speaking college or university. The minimum scores accepted are as follows: internet TOEFL = 100, paper TOEFL = 600, MELAB = 84, IELTS = 7. Please see website for additional information and deadlines.

VMCAS Participation: full

Accepts International Students? yes

Application Deadline: 9/17/2018

INTERNATIONAL
VETERINARY MEDICAL SCHOOLS
COE Accredited

ATLANTIC VETERINARY COLLEGE
AT THE UNIVERSITY OF PRINCE EDWARD ISLAND

Email Address: registrar@upei.ca

Website: www.upei.ca/programsandcourses
/professional-programs/doctor-veterinary-medicine

SCHOOL DESCRIPTION

The Atlantic Veterinary College (AVC) opened in 1986 and, since then, has graduated over 1,500 Doctors of Veterinary Medicine. It is fully accredited by the American Veterinary Medical Association and the Canadian Veterinary Medical Association, and is recognized by the Royal College of Veterinary Surgeons (UK).

Located on Canada's eastern seaboard (650 miles northeast of Boston), the Atlantic Veterinary College makes its home in beautiful Charlottetown, Prince Edward Island. With a population of just over 145,000, which jumps to over a million during the summer tourist season, Prince Edward Island is a mixture of rural and urban living, with agriculture, fishing, and tourism the mainstays of its economy. The capital city of Charlottetown (population 35,000) combines a small-town lifestyle with the amenities of larger cities, including dining and theatre. Residents also enjoy outdoor activities, such as golfing, cycling, sailing, and cross-country skiing.

> The Atlantic Veterinary College is a completely integrated teaching, research, and service facility.

The college is a completely integrated teaching, research, and service facility. The four-story complex contains the veterinary teaching hospital, diagnostic services, fish health unit, farm services, postmortem services, animal barns, laboratories, classrooms, information technology services, offices, cafeteria, and study areas.

The AVC Veterinary Teaching Hospital is the most comprehensive veterinary referral hospital in Atlantic Canada and provides care for over 6,000 animals yearly.

Students have the opportunity to work closely with faculty clinicians to manage the care and treatment of dogs, cats, horses, and cattle as well as a variety of other domestic and non-domestic species.

APPLICATION INFORMATION

For specific application information, please visit www.upei.ca/programsandcourses/professional-programs/doctor-veterinary-medicine.

Residency implications: Atlantic Veterinary College contracts with New Brunswick (13), Newfoundland (3), Nova Scotia (16), and the home province P.E.I. (10). International students are admitted on a noncontract basis (26).

SUMMARY OF ADMISSIONS PROCEDURES

Timetable

VMCAS application deadline: Monday, September 17, 2018 at 12 Midnight Eastern Time

Date international interviews are held: November

Date international acceptances mailed: January

School begins: late August

Deposit (to hold place in class): $500.00Can

Deferments: are considered on a case-by-case basis.

EVALUATION CRITERIA

Academic credentials including the GRE are evaluated by the Registrar's Office. Nonacademic ability is evaluated by the admissions committee through an interview process, a psychometric test, and review of the VMCAS application.

% weight
Academic ability 60%
Nonacademic ability 40%

ENTRANCE REQUIREMENTS

Required undergraduate GPA: no minimum stated (under review as stated above); mean cumulative GPA of most recent entering class is 3.70 on a 4.00 scale.

Is a Bachelor's Degree Required? no

Is this an International School? yes

ESTIMATED TUITION

Estimated Tuition Resident: $12,746Can (approx.)

Estimated Tuition Contract: $12,746Can (approx.)

Estimated Tuition Non-Resident: $66,500Can (equivalent to a payment of approx. $27,262US on September 15, 2017, and $26,552US on January 12, 2018)

AVAILABLE SEATS

Resident: 10

Contract: 32

Non-Resident: 26

TEST REQUIREMENTS

Standardized examinations: Graduate Record Examination (GRE). If a student's native language or language of prior education is not English, then the student will be required to submit an acceptable English Proficiency Test score.

VMCAS Participation: full

Accepts International Students? yes

ADDITIONAL INFORMATION

Application Deadline: 9/17/2018

UNIVERSITY OF CALGARY

Email Address: vet.admissions@ucalgary.ca
Website: vet.ucalgary.ca/dvmprogram

UNIVERSITY OF CALGARY
FACULTY OF VETERINARY MEDICINE

SCHOOL DESCRIPTION

The University of Calgary Faculty of Veterinary Medicine (UCVM) offers a four-year professional degree leading to a Doctor of Veterinary Medicine (DVM). Completion of at least 4 or more semesters of full-time post-secondary instruction at a recognized university or at a college providing university-equivalency in coursework is required prior to application to the DVM program.

> The University of Calgary (UCVM) offers a four-year professional degree leading to a DVM.

APPLICATION INFORMATION

Access to the online application form for the Faculty of Veterinary Medicine can be found on the website (https://vet.ucalgary.ca/dvmprogram). Applicants must be Alberta residents at the time of application, as defined by the Province of Alberta. The Alberta Government Guidelines within the Student Financial Assistance Regulations will be used to determine residency status. Details of these requirements can be found on the Alberta Government website at: https://studentaid.alberta.ca/before-you-apply/eligibility.aspx. Proof of Alberta residency will be required with your application.

Completed application forms include the following: complete personal information; a signed statement verifying Alberta residency status and verifying completion of the academic requirements; post-secondary transcripts submitted by the appropriate academic institution; a statement of work experience; and a statement of major extra-curricular activities. Official transcripts should be sent directly from the reporting institution to the UCVM Admissions Office.

English language proficiency must be demonstrated for all applicants for whom English is not their first language.

SUMMARY OF ADMISSIONS PROCEDURES

The Faculty of Veterinary Medicine accepts 30-34 DVM students per year. The Admissions Committee recommends students for admission to the program on the basis of academic and non-academic factors. Students are assessed academically on performance in their last four full undergraduate terms and in ten required courses. Selected applicants are invited for an interview where non-academic factors are assessed. On interview day, applicants are required to complete an on-site essay and participate in a series of interviews and other activities. Applicants must attend interview day at their own expense. There is no entrance exam or requirement to complete the MCAT or GRE exams.

Consistent with UCVM's mandate, preference will be given to applicants who demonstrate the attributes for successful careers in veterinary practice that support rural development and sustainability, and for careers related to our areas of emphasis. While no specific animal or veterinary-related experience is required, such experience is an asset. Understanding of the veterinary profession and animal industries relevant to the applicant's career interests is expected. This can be obtained through practical experience or through other means.

Applicants will be notified of the Admissions Committee's decision in June.

ENTRANCE REQUIREMENTS

All successful applicants are required to forward $500.00 deposit within 15 working days of notification of admission. Failure to do so may result in the position being assigned to another applicant. Such deposits will be applied to the first year's fees. An applicant who accepts a position but later rescinds his or her acceptance will forfeit the entire $500.00 deposit. Successful applicants are required to have or receive immunization for tetanus and rabies following admission.

Is a Bachelor's Degree Required? no

Is this an International School? no

ESTIMATED TUITION

Estimated Tuition Resident: ~$10,860.00 CDN

Estimated Tuition Contract: n/a

Estimated Tuition Non-Resident: n/a

VMCAS Participation: no

Accepts International Students? no

FOURTH-YEAR PROFILE: MARY RENTFROW

School you are attending
University of Florida

What has been your favorite thing about attending veterinary school so far?
My favorite thing about veterinary school has been collaborating with my peers, residents, and clinicians both in the classroom and on clinics. My class and the faculty are so much like a family that it makes it exciting to be a part of this community. The people have made this experience unforgettable and incredibly rewarding.

What advice do you have for prospective veterinary school applicants?
Get well-rounded experiences with a variety of species and to focus on building meaningful relationships with your mentors during that time. The veterinarians I shadowed or worked with during undergrad wrote my letters of recommendation, presented me with my white coat, and will be part of my graduation. Whenever I have needed any help during school, those doctors have all gone above and beyond to help me succeed. Those relationships may seem like a means to an end now, but the value of solid mentorship throughout your career cannot be understated.

What are your short-term and long-term goals?
My short-term goals are to work in small animal general practice and do relief work with emergency medicine, international wildlife campaigns, and disaster aid when possible. My long-term goals include possibly starting a business within the field or owning a practice.

What extracurricular activities are you involved in during veterinary school?
During veterinary school, I have been a member of a number of clubs and organizations, including SAVMA and the VBMA. I also acted as one of the wet lab coordinators for both surgery club and internal medicine club. Outside of school, I spent a lot of time taking classes at the gym and played intramural beach volleyball.

What was the biggest challenge you faced during veterinary school?
The biggest challenge I faced in veterinary school was trying to prioritize my time. In the beginning, I wanted to be actively involved in every organization on campus while also working part time. I realized I had to prioritize what I was most passionate about to really get the most out of school.

What advice do you have for other students who are currently in veterinary school?
My advice would be to support each other throughout these four years. No one else understands the stress of school better than your classmates. Also, don't spend all of your time studying. It is definitely important and vital to your success, but burnout is a real problem in veterinary medicine. Creating good habits and striving for a healthy work-life balance now will better prepare you to have a sustainable career later in life.

Why do you want to be a veterinarian?
I want to be a veterinarian because I find it both challenging and exciting. Each case requires you to think critically and empathetically. Most importantly, every day you get the chance to save lives and help not only the animals, but also their humans.

What field of veterinary medicine are you interested in pursuing and why?
I am most interested in a career in small animal general practice because I love building lasting relationships with clients and patients. I also enjoy doing a little bit of everything when it comes to medicine, surgery, cardiology, anesthesia, and so forth, and general practice allows me to do that. I have a passion for exotics, as well, and I hope to volunteer abroad in the future.

UNIVERSITY COLLEGE DUBLIN

Email: vetadmissions@ucd.ie
Website: www.ucd.ie/vetmed
Phone: +353 1 7166100

SCHOOL DESCRIPTION

UCD School of Veterinary Medicine is the sole provider of a veterinary medicine degree programme on the island of Ireland, and is one of only six European veterinary schools that are accredited by the American Veterinary Medical Association.

Students of the veterinary medicine programme benefit from the outstanding facilities of the purpose-designed UCD Veterinary Sciences Centre and UCD Veterinary Hospital on the main university campus at Belfield, Dublin (commissioned in 2002). Located on a 132 Ha site 5km south of Dublin's City Centre, UCD is Ireland's largest university with over 30,000 students. This is complemented by Lyons Estate Farm where students have practical classes at all stages of the curriculum.

> The programme is designed to educate you to the best international standards in veterinary medicine.

As the gateway to Europe, Ireland has been renowned for learning and creativity for centuries. Our English-speaking, well-educated population has drawn global companies like Google, Facebook, Intel and HP, who now collaborate with us and employ our graduates.

With its unique blend of urban chic, lush parkland, sweeping coastline, fabulous shopping and excellent cultural experiences, Dublin is without a doubt one of the most energised capital cities in Europe.

UCD is a diverse, international campus. Our student population comprises of more than 50 nationalities, and international students now account for one-third of the total undergraduate student cohort. This diversity is one of the defining features of life at UCD, and one that enriches the student experience by provision of a truly international campus. Your experience as a vet student at UCD will guarantee life-long friendships. You can find further information on attending UCD as an international student at http://www.ucd.ie/international.

Programme/Syllabus

Our veterinary programme is accredited by the Veterinary Council of Ireland, the American Veterinary Medical Association, and the European Association of Establishments in Veterinary Education. It is designed to educate you to the best international standards in veterinary medicine and to prepare you for entry to any branch of the veterinary profession. Veterinary medicine is concerned with the promotion of the health and welfare of animals of special importance to society. This involves the care for healthy and sick animals, the prevention, recognition, control and treatment of their diseases and the welfare and productivity of livestock. Veterinarians also safeguard human health through prevention and control of diseases transmitted from animals to man, through ensuring the safety of foods of animal origin, and through advancing the science and art of comparative medicine.

Veterinary graduates have a wide spectrum of careers to choose from including private practice (companion animals, food animals, horses, exotics, or a mixture of these), government service (animal health, food safety, public health), research or industry.

US applicants through VMCAS are eligible to apply to enter this programme provided they have the prerequisites as outlined below. Further curricular details are published on our web site, www.ucd.ie/vetmed.

PREREQUISITES FOR ADMISSION

4-Year Graduate-Entry Programme

Candidates who have studied and will complete a degree in an appropriate biological science may be considered for the 4-year Graduate programme in Veterinary Medicine with the award of MVB.

Course Requirements	Full Semester
Physics with lab	1
Biochemistry	1
General biology	1
General inorganic chemistry with lab	1
Microbiology	1
Cellular biology	1

Course completion deadline: all required courses should be completed prior to August of the year of admission.

5-Year Undergraduate Programme MVB

Those candidates with a non-science degree or lacking some prerequisites or sufficient relevant experience will be considered entry to the 5-year MVB programme.

Standardized examinations: none required. GRE results will be considered if submitted.

Additional requirements and considerations

A minimum of two references must be provided (one from an academic source, and one from a practicing veterinary surgeon).

Applicants are expected to have gained relevant work experience of handling animals. This should, where possible, include not only seeing veterinary practice, but also spending time on livestock farms and other animal establishments.

The Graduate-Entry Programme is organised into four stages. In stage 1 of the programme students will build on their knowledge of the basic biological sciences by taking modules designed to demonstrate how this knowledge is applied in the practice of veterinary medicine, and gain a firm grounding in animal welfare, behaviour and handling. A key objective will be to ensure that students have the required knowledge, skills and competences to progress to Stage 2. Starting with stage 2 students will take modules with students of the five year undergraduate veterinary medicine programme. As the programme progresses students will learn clinical skills and study each of the clinical sciences using a "body systems" approach. The final year of the programme consists of clinical rotations in the UCD teaching hospital where students have the opportunity to work alongside experienced and specialist staff clinicians, and participate in patient care and client communication. Each student has a personalized timetable ensuring that they participate in rotations in Large and Small Animal Surgery, Diagnostic Imaging, Anesthesiology, Small Animal Medicine, Emergency Medicine, Farm Animal Clinical Studies including Herd Health, Diagnostic and Clinical Pathology, as well as a rotation in shelter medicine, which is provided in collaboration with the Dublin Society for the Prevention of Cruelty to Animals (DSPCA). Throughout the programme students are required to participate in extra-mural studies. In the early years, this consists of gaining experience in the handling and management of farm and companion animals, and in later years, of working with veterinarians in practice (clinical extra-mural experience).

APPLICATION INFORMATION

UCD is participating in the VMCAS application system. A supplemental application through the UCD online application system is required.

Fees for non-EU students for entry to the 4 year programme in 2017 were €36,300 per annum. Fees for non-EU students for entry to the 5 year programme in 2017 were €30,700 per annum. For further information on entry to the Republic of Ireland, please refer to www.educationireland.com.

SUMMARY OF ADMISSION PROCEDURE

Timetable

VMCAS application deadline: Monday, September 17, 2018 at 12 Midnight Eastern Time

Supplemental application deadline: November 1, 2018

Interviews: January/February (held in the US)

Date acceptances mailed: early April

Deposit (to hold place in class): €2,000, required within 2 weeks of acceptance

Deferments: Not applicable

EVALUATION CRITERIA INCLUDE

Academic performance (a minimum GPA of 3.2 is required)

References/evaluations (minimum 2 required-one from academic science source and one from a practicing veterinary surgeon)

1-page personal statement

Record of Animal and Veterinary Experience

Interview

ESTIMATED TUITION

Resident/Sponsored: €20,300
Non-Resident: €36,300

AVAILABLE SEATS

Resident: 90
Non-Resident: 35

ADMISSION PROCESS

US and Canadian residents must apply to UCD through VMCAS and a supplemental application form which is available at www.ucd.ie/vetmed.

Completed applications are reviewed by our admissions team. Successful applicants will receive their offers from December onwards. Classes begin in early September with compulsory orientation taking place prior to the start of classes.

* For up-to-date information on fees and all further information regarding admission to University College Dublin, please visit our web site www.ucd.ie.

UNIVERSITY OF EDINBURGH

Email Address: vetug@ed.ac.uk
Website: www.ed.ac.uk/vet

SCHOOL DESCRIPTION

The Royal (Dick) School of Veterinary Studies was founded by William Dick in 1823, and sits within the College of Medicine and Veterinary Medicine at the University of Edinburgh. The School is a recognized world leader in veterinary education, research and clinical practice. The BVM&S degree is accredited by the Royal College of Veterinary Surgeons (RCVS), the American Veterinary Medical Association (AVMA), the Australasian Veterinary Boards Council (AVBC), the South African Veterinary Council (SAVC), and the European Association of Establishments for Veterinary Education (EAEVE), allowing our graduates to practice veterinary medicine throughout the United Kingdom, North America, Europe, Australasia and beyond.

> The School is a recognized world leader in veterinary education, research and clinical practice.

Veterinary Medicine at Edinburgh mixes the best of tradition with award winning, progressive teaching. Clinical and professional skills are taught from the earliest stages. Our approach is to ensure optimum integration of the core subjects throughout the curriculum. While many of our graduates enter and remain within the veterinary profession, many others find that training at Edinburgh enables them to succeed in a wide range of careers in research, government, private enterprise and academia.

The Easter Bush campus houses the Royal (Dick) School of Veterinary Studies which incorporates The Roslin Institute, Jeanne Marchig International Centre for Animal Welfare Education and the Veterinary Oncology and Imaging Centre. The Roslin Institute (now the research arm of the Veterinary School) is an animal sciences research institute, which won international fame in 1996, when Ian Wilmut, Keith Campbell and their colleagues created Dolly the sheep, the first mammal to be cloned from an adult cell.

Within the University of Edinburgh, there are over 260 student societies – more than any other university in the UK – covering everything from juggling to horse riding to volunteering, which can cater to your interests. Our sports, music and drama facilities are ranked among the best in the UK.

Edinburgh, the inspiring capital of Scotland, is an historic, cosmopolitan and cultured city, which offers a unique living and learning experience. One of the most vibrant cities in Europe, the city of Edinburgh is regularly voted as one of the most desirable places to live in the world and has been rated the "friendliest city in the UK." This cosmopolitan, safe and welcoming atmosphere encourages all students to feel at home very quickly. With a population of around 500,000, Edinburgh is a compact city, which is easy to travel around on foot or by the efficient public transport network. Edinburgh International Airport has an extensive range of national and international services with direct flights to most major cities in Europe and to a number of major cities worldwide. Many students also take the opportunity to travel around Europe during vacation periods, or even for the weekend, as there are many cheap flight options available from Edinburgh.

For more information on our Veterinary Medicine and Surgery degree programs, refer to the following link: www.ed.ac.uk/schools-departments/vet/studying/bvms-degree.

APPLICATION INFORMATION

For specific application information on availability, key deadlines, fees, VMCAS participation and more, refer to the following link www.ed.ac.uk/schools-departments /vet/studying/bvms-degree alternatively feel free to contact us directly by email at vetug@ed.ac.uk.

Residency implications: For full details and further information on entry to the UK, please refer to https:// www.gov.uk/government/organisations/uk-visas-and -immigration. Please note that students must be able to ensure adequate financial support for the duration of their course.

SUMMARY OF ADMISSIONS PROCEDURES

Timetable

VMCAS application deadline: Monday, September 17, 2018 at 12 Midnight Eastern Time

GRE scores deadline: October 1, 2018 at 12 Midnight Eastern Time

Interviews: early to mid-February (held in the U.S.)

Date acceptances mailed: early April at the latest

School begins: early August (4-year Graduate Entry Program), early September (5-year program)

Deposit (to hold place in class): £1,500, required by early May

Deferments: Not applicable. Candidates are not required to submit a supplemental application.

Full details of Edinburgh's application calendar is available here: http://www.ed.ac.uk/schools-departments/vet /studying/overview

EVALUATION CRITERIA

Academic performance

GRE scores

Animal/veterinary experience

Personal statement

Motivation

References/Evaluations (minimum 2 required—one from academic science source and one from a veterinary surgeon)

Interview

ENTRANCE REQUIREMENTS

Graduate Entry (Undergraduate degree-holders or in senior year of degree)

Candidates with a degree (or in their senior year) in an appropriate Biological or Animal Science degree may be considered for the 4-year BVM&S program (Graduate Entry Program). All applicants are required to have completed the required prerequisite courses for the program to a high standard. US applicants should have an overall minimum grade point average of 3.4 (4 point scale), with greater than 3.0 in science courses. The School also welcomes applications from candidates with an alternative degree who have also completed the required prerequisites to a high standard. Candidates with a non-science degree would normally be considered for the 5-year BVM&S program. However, if candidates have the specified prerequisites, they may be considered for the 4-year program.

Pre-Vet

Candidates with two years of a pre-vet will be considered for the 5-year BVM&S program. An overall GPA of 3.4 (4 point scale) is expected. All applicants are required to have completed the required prerequisite courses for the program.

Further information about Edinburgh's prerequisites for the BVM&S program is available here: http://www .ed.ac.uk/schools-departments/vet/studying/bvms -degree

Is a Bachelor's Degree Required? yes (4-year GEP), no (5-year)

Is this an International School? yes

ESTIMATED TUITION

Estimated Tuition Non-Resident: £30,800 per annum, fixed for the duration of the program

AVAILABLE SEATS

Resident: 72

Non-Resident: 98

TEST REQUIREMENTS

Standardized examinations: Graduate Record Examination (GRE) general test is required. The scores must be received by October 1 for 2019 entry. Applicants should ensure they take the GRE early enough for scores to be received before the deadline.

Note that the following tests are NOT required for candidates applying to the BVM&S programs at the University of Edinburgh:

- BioMedical Admissions Test (BMAT)
- UK Clinical Aptitude Test (UKCAT)
- Medical College Admission Test (MCAT)
- Veterinary College Admission Test (VCAT)

VMCAS Participation: partial

Accepts International Students? yes

ADDITIONAL INFORMATION

For up-to-date information on fees and all further information regarding admission to the School, please visit our website http://www.ed.ac.uk/schools-departments/vet

UNIVERSITY OF GLASGOW

Email Address: vet-sch-admissions@glasgow.ac.uk
Website: http://www.gla.ac.uk/schools/vet

SCHOOL DESCRIPTION

The School of Veterinary Medicine is located on the 80 hectare Garscube campus at the Northwest boundary of the city, four miles from the University's Gilmorehill campus. The School was founded in 1862 and gained independent Faculty status in 1969. In 2010, the Faculty translated from the "Faculty of Veterinary Medicine" to the "School of Veterinary Medicine" within the College of Medical, Veterinary and Life Sciences.

> The BVMS programme is based on integration of clinical and science subject areas and has a spiral course structure.

The School has a 190 hectare commercial farm and research centre at Cochno, 15 minutes from the Garscube campus (5 miles north).

The city of Glasgow has a population of around 600,000 and is Scotland's largest city. One of Europe's liveliest places with a varied and colorful cultural and social life, it can cater to every taste. Situated on the River Clyde, Glasgow has excellent road and rail links to the rest of the UK and air services to a wide range of destinations, both home and overseas.

Wherever you come from, you can be sure of building friendships that last a lifetime at Glasgow. According to travel guide Lonely Planet, Glasgow is one of the world's top ten cities.

The School has approximately 200 staff (academic, research, and support) with an additional 65 postgraduate research students, 30 postgraduate clinical scholars, and 600 undergraduate students.

The school is pre-eminent in teaching, research, and clinical provision, and attracts students, researchers, and clinicians from around the world. Our internationally accredited school provides an expert referral centre via the Small Animal Hospital, the Weipers Centre for Equine Welfare, and the Scottish Centre for Production Animal Health & Welfare for animal owners and referring practitioners throughout the UK.

Following the first ever international UK accreditation visit to be undertaken conjointly between the American Veterinary Medical Association (AVMA) Council on Education, the Royal College of Veterinary Surgeons (RCVS), the European Association of Establishments for Veterinary Education (EAEVE), and the Australasian Veterinary Boards Council (AVBC) in April 2013, the University of Glasgow's School of Veterinary Medicine has achieved full accreditation for a further period of seven years.

The BVMS programme is based on integration of clinical and science subject areas and has a spiral course structure, meaning that you will revisit topics as you progress through the programme, each time with increasing clinical focus. In conjunction, there is a vertical theme of professional and clinical skills development to help you acquire the personal qualities and skills you will need in professional environments.

The programme is delivered over five years and is divided into three phases. Years 1 and 2, Foundation Phase, Years 3 and 5, Clinical Phase, Year 5, Professional Phase.

In the recent Research Excellence Framework 2014 (REF2014), the Grade Point Average for Glasgow's veterinary and animal health research activity was ranked top amongst the UK veterinary schools.

EXTRAMURAL STUDIES

In common with all veterinary students in the UK, you will be required to undertake an additional 38 weeks of extra-mural studies (EMS) during your vacation time. The first period of 12 weeks is dedicated to gaining further experience of the management and handling of domestic animals. After this initial period is completed, you start the clinical period of 26 weeks, which can be used to gain experience in veterinary professional environments. Satisfactory completion of EMS is a requirement for graduation.

APPLICATION INFORMATION

For specific application information (availability, deadlines, fees, and VMCAS participation), please refer to the contact information listed above.

Residency implications: Due to recent changes in immigration legislation, students from the U.S. (who are planning to come to the UK for more than 6 months) are now required to obtain an entry clearance certificate prior to entering the UK. For further information on entry to the UK, please refer to https://www.gov.uk/tier-4-general-visa. Students must also be able to ensure adequate financial support for the duration of their course.

SUMMARY OF ADMISSIONS PROCEDURES

Timetable

VMCAS application deadline: Monday, September 17, 2018 at 12 Midnight Eastern Time

Date interviews held: November-February (In the U.S. and Canada)

Date acceptances mailed: April

School begins: late September

Deposit (to hold place in class): £1,000

Deferments: in certain circumstances

EVALUATION CRITERIA

Academic performance
Animal/veterinary experience
References
Essay
Interview
Entrance Requirements
Course requirements
 Applicants are expected to have completed at least 2 years Pre-Veterinary or science courses at College or University, with a minimum of one year in chemistry (including organic chemistry and organic chem-istry lab), biology, or biochemistry, and either physics, maths, or statistics. We would expect high grades in all science subjects. US applicant should have a minimum 3.4 GPA (4 point scale), and to have achieved at 3.0 in Science.

Required undergraduate GPA: 3.40

AP credit policy: not applicable

Course completion deadline: required courses should be completed prior to admission in the fall.

Standardized examinations: none required. GRE results will be considered if submitted.

ADDITIONAL REQUIREMENTS AND CONSIDERATIONS

Animal/veterinary work experience sufficient to indicate motivation, interest, and understanding of the veterinary profession
 Evaluations: minimum 2, one each from an academic science source and a veterinary surgeon.
 There is no supplemental application for the University of Glasgow.

Is a Bachelor's Degree Required? no

Is this an International School? yes

ESTIMATED TUITION

Resident of UK out with Scotland: £9,250/yr

International: £29,250 (fixed at the point of entry). Fees are set in UK Sterling, and there will be a fluctuation in the exchange rate.

AVAILABLE SEATS

Resident: 72

Non-Resident: 60

TEST REQUIREMENTS

Standardized examinations: none required. GRE results will be considered if submitted.

VMCAS Participation: partial

Accepts International Students? yes

ADDITIONAL INFORMATION

For further information, contact the Undergraduate School Admissions Office (vet-sch-admissions@glasgow.ac.uk)

Application Deadline: 9/17/2018

UNIVERSITY OF GUELPH

Email: vetmed@uoguelph.ca
Website: www.ovc.uoguelph.ca/ recruitment/en
/index.asp

ONTARIO
VETERINARY COLLEGE

SCHOOL DESCRIPTION

The Ontario Veterinary College (OVC) at the University of Guelph is a world leader in veterinary health care, learning and research. We work at the intersection of animal, human, and ecosystem health.

Founded in 1862, OVC is the oldest veterinary school in Canada and the United States. OVC is located in Ontario, at the University of Guelph, and is a short drive from one of Canada's largest and well-known hubs of activity and culture, Toronto. A drive north takes you to the first of Canada's many popular lakes, known for clear waters and havens of nature.

> The Ontario Veterinary College works at the intersection of animal, human, and ecosystem health.

Academically, OVC is consistently ranked as one of Canada's top universities. In fact, we're renowned worldwide for excellence in teaching, research and service, with graduates of the program practicing veterinary medicine, conducting research or working in related industry across the globe.

With faculty and administration sharing like-minded ideas on furthering animal care, research and innovative teaching methodologies, OVC offers a rich and intense learning environment to students. Our health sciences centre and facilities specialize in large and small animals, with dedicated intensive, primary, and oncology care, mean the potential for hands-on and applied learning are endless.

Researchers at OVC conduct innovative, collaborative research aimed at improving the health and well-being of animals, humans, and ecosystems. This work covers a broad scope of disciplines ranging from basic laboratory investigation, to epidemiological field studies, to applied clinical research on companion and food animals as well as wildlife. Research at OVC is performed within a framework of the following guiding principles: Excellence, Uniqueness, Collaboration, Innovation, Communication, and Training.

DVM students can work on summer research projects with OVC faculty and participate in our Summer Career Opportunities and Research Exploration Program.

One of five veterinary colleges in Canada, OVC is accredited by the American Veterinary Medical Association, Canadian and American Medical Associations and the Royal College of Veterinary Surgeons of the United Kingdom. OVC grads can be licensed in these countries, giving graduates a spectrum of opportunities.

APPLICATION INFORMATION

Each year, the Ontario Veterinary College (OVC) accepts up to 15 U.S. and international (non-Canadian) students. This year, you could be one of those students!

International applicants must not hold Canadian citizenship (this includes dual citizenship) or Permanent Resident status. Students can apply as early as the summer after their sophomore year provided they have a GPA of 3.2 or above and have completed the prerequisite courses.

PREREQUISITES FOR ADMISSION	
Course Description	**Number of Hours/Credits**
3 Biological Sciences (1 with Cell Biology content)	9
Biochemistry	3
Statistics	3
Genetics	3
Humanities/Social Science*	6

*Consider topics such as ethics, logic, critical thinking, determinants of human behaviour and human social interaction.

Applicants who receive an offer of admission should be aware that they must meet federal immigration requirements for entry into Canada as a student.

Non-Canadian applicants who have fulfilled the academic requirements for the Doctor of Veterinary Medicine (DVM) program should apply using the Veterinary Medical College Application Service (VMCAS).

SUMMARY OF ADMISSIONS PROCEDURES

Checklist for non-Canadians applying to the University of Guelph DVM program

Note: if you hold dual Canadian citizenship you MUST apply as a Canadian.

Pre-Application

Complete 2 years of university and the 8 prerequisites within full-time semesters.

Application (September)

Veterinary Medical College Application Service (VMCAS) online application including:

- 3 referee assessments (from 2 veterinarians and 1 professional)

- Background information

- Application fee (to VMCAS)

- The Academic Background form must be submitted separately: http://www.ovc.uoguelph.ca/recruitment/en/applyingtodvm/resources/Prerequisiteform.pdf

- If you are already attending or have attended the University of Guelph please apply using the Application for Internal Transfer/Readmission Form.

Information is gathered through the Academic Background Form (ABF), References, and Transcripts.

November

- Academic Background Form with Course Descriptions (syllabus)
- Supplemental fee

You will be assigned a University of Guelph email account with which you can access your WebAdvisor account for updates on your application status.

November-July

If selected for an interview, you will be contacted by email. Interviews are 45 minutes long with two members of faculty and are usually held at the Ontario Veterinary College in Guelph. Virtual interviews using Skype are offered for those who cannot visit us in person.

On the day of your on-site interview you will be provided with a tour of the college led by a current DVM student.

Applicants can monitor the status of their application on their University of Guelph WebAdvisor account. Applicants will then be notified by email and letter of the final decision regarding their application.

*Application directly to the University of Guelph is also available and forms can be obtained by emailing vetmed@uoguelph.ca

If you have questions about the application procedure or a current application in progress, please contact:

Kelly Hunter, Admission Services
519-824-4120 Ext. 58711

ENTRANCE REQUIREMENTS

College/University

Complete at least two years (4 semesters) of full-time studies in an accredited college or university. Full-time is usually 12 credit hours at a US school.

All prerequisite courses can be completed in any year of their post-secondary studies. Courses should be completed within a college or university undergraduate program. Courses taken during professional programs or certificate/technical programs are not acceptable.

Students from the US should take a minimum of 12.00 credit hours per semester. Courses must be taken/studied at the same time to ensure an appropriate work load. Field courses or any courses that are pursued over one semester and credited in another semester do not count towards the latter semester's courses for this purpose.

You can study at any accredited college or university and take any major that interests you. You can apply to the DVM program after completing two years of university. If accepted, you do not need to finish your four-year degree program and can simply transfer to the DVM program.

A course that runs the full year will have the credit weight divided equally and half applied to each of the two semesters the course is taken.

Please note that the GPA from your last two full-time semesters, and the average from your 8 prerequisite courses must both be 3.2 on a 4 point scale or higher in order for you to be considered further for entry to the DVM program.

Important Regulations Regarding Acceptable Courses

Only prerequisite courses must be completed at the college/university level before admission to the Doctor of Veterinary Medicine Program will be considered. Courses do not need to be completed in a designated Pre-Veterinary program.

Courses will not be acceptable if they are repeats of previously passed courses, or if they are taken at the same level or a lower level in a subject area if they have significant overlap of content. Students should consider their institution's course sequencing in determining if a course is considered the same level.

The DVM Admissions Committee cannot evaluate Honours, Pass-Fail, and Satisfactory-Unsatisfactory grading systems. Applicants should obtain a numerical or letter grade for all required courses and the grades should be certified by the Registrar of the university attended.

Candidates who hold a non-science bachelor's degree in which they did not take some of the prerequisite courses because they were not part of their program may return to university as part of a non-degree semester(s) to gain the prerequisites. These courses must be assessed by the University of Guelph Admissions Office for content.

Failure to comply with the course level rules will result in the exclusion of all coursework from the ineligible semester(s) toward a DVM application.

Course Evaluation Request

If you are not studying at the University of Guelph, you must submit up to two options for the courses that you want to use as prerequisites for approval prior to application.

Requests must include:

- A transcript of university courses completed to date—a photocopy is fine. Please know that some schools report courses by year only on their transcripts, so a breakdown of which were done in which semesters must also be included.

- A list of proposed courses for any future semesters you are planning. Be sure to break down your proposed courses by semester. We cannot assess by year.

- A list of the eight courses to be presented as prerequisite courses and detailed course descriptions for each. You may present one or two choices (no more) for each of the eight. Do not submit full syllabi with your request. If further information is required, we will contact you. Please ensure to include course codes, pre/anti-requisites, course titles and clearly identify which course is being presented as which prerequisite. Word or PDF documents are preferred.

- A maximum of two attachments: one for the course evaluation and one for your transcript. If you have attended multiple institutions, you may include additional attachments.

- Your email address and contact information.

Please email the information to admdvm@uoguelph .ca; indicate Course Evaluation Request with your name in the Subject line. You will be sent an email confirming the receipt of your course evaluation request.

Further instructions can be found on our website: http://www.ovc.uoguelph.ca/recruitment/en/applying todvm/Academicrequirements.asp

Individuals wishing to appeal decisions related to admissions eligibility may submit a letter detailing their individual circumstance and any letters/documentation of support to:

Chair, Admissions Committee,
  Ontario Veterinary College
c/o Kelly Hunter

Admission Services UC L3
University of Guelph
Guelph, ON N1G 2W1
Fax: 519-766-9481
email: admdvm@uoguelph.ca

Please note that appeals are due March 1 of the year of application, and submitting an appeal in no way guarantees a positive response.

NON-ACADEMIC REQUIREMENTS

Veterinary experience
Veterinary experience may be voluntary or paid, but must be done with a supervising veterinarian in placements such as clinical practice, research laboratories, animal shelters, animal rehabilitation facilities, public health settings or another related industry where a veterinarian is employed.

Although there is no minimum required number of hours needed for application, it is strongly advised that applicants log as many hours as possible. Try working with different species, too, such as swine, cows, horses, exotics, dogs, cats, etc. Experience within Canada and the USA is recommended.

Animal experience
Animal experience includes working with livestock, breeding/showing various species, working in a pet store, equestrian activities and any other animal related hobby/experience where a veterinarian is not always present, or does not supervise you. Animal experience does not include pet ownership. Animals are defined as vertebrates for this purpose.

Extracurricular experience
So much of veterinary medicine involves working with people and as part of a service team. Jobs and volunteer activities that hone your communication, interpersonal and organizational skills are important. These experiences do not involve animal contact.

Referee assessments
Three only confidential referee assessments comprised of an evaluative grid and a letter are required for each DVM applicant.

The referees must be qualified to give an unbiased, informed and critical assessment of the applicant. Two of the three referees selected must be veterinarians with whom he or she has obtained veterinary and/or animal experience. There is a strong preference for veterinarians from different clinics or workplaces and may include DVMs in such areas as government, industry, and research. The goal of having the veterinary references is to have those within the profession assess whether you are a suitable candidate to join that profession, therefore it is important that the referees understand what is required of veterinarians in a Canadian/US context.

None of your references should be from family members, long standing friends, or your colleagues or colleagues of your family, even if they are veterinarians. These are not considered objective sources. Your referees should be individuals who know you in a supervisory or professional context and are able to assess you objectively. Applications from candidates with referee assessments from family, colleagues or friends will not be considered suitable for further consideration and will not be invited for an interview.

Graduate students (those from masters or doctoral degree programs) may request an additional form to highlight their accomplishments while within their graduate program.

Is a Bachelor's Degree Required? no

Is this an International School? yes

ESTIMATED TUITION

Estimated Tuition Resident: n/a

Estimated Tuition Contract: n/a

Estimated Tuition Non-Resident: $61,330 Canadian Funds per year

AVAILABLE SEATS

Resident: 105

Contract: n/a

Non-Resident (International): 15

TEST REQUIREMENTS

None

VMCAS Participation: full

Accepts International Students? yes

ADDITIONAL INFORMATION

Application Deadline: 9/17/2018

PRE-VETERINARY PROFILE: SAMANTHA LARKIN

Current School Name
Juniata College

What type of veterinary medicine are you interested in pursuing, and why?
I have a particular interest in wildlife medicine and exotic animals. I have always had a passion for exotics and wildlife, and I think I will enjoy the challenge of working with different animals.

What is/was your major during undergraduate school?
Zoology.

What are your short-term and long-term goals?
I have multiple short-term goals. Since I am a senior in college, the most immediate goals concern the gap year that I plan to take. I am seeking jobs or volunteer opportunities with wildlife for this time. I am also attempting to put together my application for veterinary school. My next goals concern getting into vet school and doing well, and then studying a specialty. My ultimate long-term goal is to dedicate myself to helping endangered species; however, I am very open to the possibility of my goals changing as I learn more and go through veterinary school.

What are you doing as an applicant/pre-vet to prepare for veterinary school?
During college, I have worked to get all the prerequisites, grades, and opportunities to gain hours for my application to be considered. I also researched schools this summer to ensure I had all the prerequisites for the schools to which I may want to apply. I am currently working on putting my application together. I took a class during the fall semester of my senior year that gets the application process started. We are asked to write our personal statement and to outline all of our experiences and explain why they are meaningful to help with our application.

What extracurricular activities are you involved in currently?
I am an officer of the Tri-Beta organization (biology honor society) at my college; a member of concert band; an officer in the equestrian club; a student assistant in Academic Support; and a tutor for chemistry, biostatistics, and vertebrate zoology.

How old were you when you first became interested in being a veterinarian?
I was very young when I found my passion for animals. I love to help people and animals alike, so I have wanted to be a veterinarian for most of my life. I have considered other careers, and during certain times I have been unsure if this was truly the path I wanted to pursue. However, looking into other careers always seemed to solidify my desire to be a veterinarian.

Please describe your various experiences in preparation for applying to veterinary school.
I started working at a horse farm my senior year of high school and I continued to work there the summer I got home from college to gain experience working with animals other than dogs and cats. I also did some limited shadowing over the summer between my freshman and sophomore year of college. My junior year, I shadowed veterinarians one day a week during the fall. I had the opportunity to participate in an EPA program where I worked 20 hours a week in a veterinary practice for four months in London. When I came home, I was able to get a job at a veterinary physical therapy facility for the summer as a veterinary technician.

What characteristics are you looking for in a veterinary school?
I am looking for a school with opportunities to work with various animals in different disciplines. I hope to find one that offers opportunities to work with wildlife and exotic animals in particular. I also hope to attend a school where most of the learning is hands-on.

What advice do you have for other pre-veterinary students?
You should get as much experience as possible, but try to take care of yourself. You should work hard to get the grades and find opportunities to work with animals whenever possible, but also find your interests and follow them. Don't be afraid to try new things. The veterinary field is larger than most people imagine; there are so many specialties to discover and shadow if you look for the opportunities.

MASSEY UNIVERSITY

Email Address: vetschool@massey.ac.nz
Website: www.massey.ac.nz/vetschool

MASSEY
VETERINARY
SCHOOL

WHY MASSEY UNIVERSITY?

The Massey University veterinary program was the first veterinary program to gain AVMA accreditation in the southern hemisphere. Our program is also fully accredited by the Australasian Veterinary Board Council (AVBC), the Royal College of Veterinary Surgeons (RCVS) and is recognised through reciprocity by the South African Veterinary Association (SAVA). This means you could work as a veterinarian not only in the USA and Canada, but also New Zealand, Australia, the United Kingdom, and many other countries.

> The Massey University veterinary school staff are collegial, motivated, highly qualified individuals.

The Massey University veterinary program has an international reputation for providing an excellent veterinary education with a strong science background, a broad knowledge of companion, equine, and production animal health, and a focus on independent thinking and problem-solving skills. So you can be sure that as a Massey graduate you'll be well prepared for your veterinary career. In fact, we've been ranked number 1 for reputation with employers and 15th programme overall in the QS rankings of veterinary programmes globally. The QS ranking is currently the only ranking system of veterinary programs around the world (including North America).

JOINING THE MASSEY VETERINARY PROGRAM

We accept up to 24 international students annually, with a total class size of 124. Our veterinary program is 5 years (10 semesters) in length, split into a "pre-selection" phase (one semester—beginning in February annually), and the "professional" phase (the remaining 9 semesters or 4.5 years). In the pre-selection phase students compete for entry into the professional phase.

As an international student, you could join our program in one of two ways depending upon your academic background.

Group 2 - Professional phase entry for international students
Group 2 students apply for entry directly into the professional phase on the basis of their academic performance overseas. You need to have completed at least two years full-time or the equivalent of an appropriate undergraduate degree. Students selected via this method would start in the professional phase in mid-July (semester 2). See the section on entrance requirements for more information.

Group 1 - Pre-selection phase entry for international students
Group 1 international students are those who do not meet all of the eligibility criteria for Group 2, or do but were not selected for a Group 2 position. Group 1 students come to New Zealand and complete the pre-selection phase in order to prove their capability for the professional phase. This is a great option for those who want to get into an AVMA accredited veterinary program who may not be the "traditional applicant."

WHAT IS THE CURRICULUM LIKE?

Throughout years 1-4 you will study core medical sciences (tailored for veterinary students), as well as normal and then abnormal animal structure and function. Then you'll be taught how to "fix" animals, or return them to normal function through clinical studies, medicine, surgery, and health management of companion and agricultural animal species.

A revised curriculum was introduced in 2013 to further increase your learning and understanding by integrating topics within and between years, and introducing problem oriented learning throughout the curriculum. This encourages students to apply the information learned in the various classes to veterinary cases and scenarios designed to develop problem solving and critical thinking. Additionally a greater emphasis has been placed on professional studies, to further enhance your future career success.

The fifth year is a semi-tracked clinically based year. You would choose a track from the following options: small animal, production animal, equine or mixed animal, or other areas as approved (e.g., wildlife, research). All tracks share a core of 18 weeks of rotations covering multiple species, then depending on which track you choose, you will have a further 7-9 weeks specified. You then have 7-9 weeks where you can choose to do externships (within New Zealand or overseas), or further clinics at Massey University. The semi-tracked, individualized final year curriculum allows you to further explore your area of interest while ensuring wide coverage of the main veterinary species.

During the programme, you will attend lectures, tutorials, practical classes, field trips, and clinical sessions and rotations, and you will also undertake farm and veterinary practical work outside of university semester time.

WHERE IS MASSEY UNIVERSITY?

The veterinary school is located in Palmerston North, a student-friendly town of 85,000 in the lower North Island of New Zealand. Palmerston North is a one-hour flight from Auckland, is conveniently close to west coast beaches, and is just under a two-hour drive to the Hawke's Bay wine region, skiing and snowboarding at Mt. Ruapehu and the capital city, Wellington. Nicknamed "student city," Palmerston North offers free bus services for Massey students and has lots of great cafés, restaurants, bars, and outdoor recreational activities.

Renowned for an excellent lifestyle, New Zealand is a great place to study abroad for your AVMA accredited veterinary degree.

APPLICATION INFORMATION

You can find more specific information (deadlines, fees, VMCAS participation, the supplemental application and direct application) on the Massey University veterinary school website.

If you are a US or Canadian resident you can apply to Massey University by either:
1. VMCAS and a supplemental Massey University application or
2. Direct application to Massey University.

All other non-New Zealand residents are to apply directly to Massey University

Residency implications: All non-New Zealand resident students require a student visa, which is easily obtained following an offer of admission into the program. A requirement for a visa is that students must be able to demonstrate financial support for the duration of their course (e.g. Federal Aid loan approval).

SUMMARY OF ADMISSIONS PROCEDURES

Timetable

Group 1

Application deadline: November 1, 2018

Letters of admission to pre-selection (semester 1) sent: Once completed application reviewed.

Pre-selection phase of school begins: Late February 2019 (semester 1)

Acceptances into the professional phase of the veterinary degree program notified: Early July 2019

Professional phase of veterinary program begins: Mid-July 2019 (semester 2)

Group 2

VMCAS application deadline: Monday, September 17, 2018 at 11:59 PM Eastern Time. Online Massey University supplemental application with all supplementary documents to be received by November 1, 2018. **Please note**, your application will not be considered until you complete your Massey University supplemental application.

Direct applicants: November 1, 2018 (including all supplementary documents)

Date acceptances mailed: from late December 2018

Professional phase of veterinary program begins: Mid-July 2019 (semester 2)

Deposit (to hold Group 2 position): $NZ 1,500.00 (non-refundable)

Deferments: Deferments of Group 1 offers (into the pre-selection phase - semester 1 of the program) are permitted. Offers of a place in semester 2 of the program are for a single year only and as such deferments are not permitted.

EVALUATION CRITERIA

Group 1

The selection process for Group 1 students is based 50% on academic performance and 50% on non-academic performance. Please see the website for more detail.

Group 2

Science GPA: 50%

Non-academic criteria: 50%
- This will include an interview

ENTRANCE REQUIREMENTS

Course requirements

Group 1: As a Group 1 applicant you would come to Massey University in late February to complete a semester of full-time science study in order to develop a GPA for selection. You would take the four prerequisite classes, or if you're given credit for these based on previous study, you'll choose alternate science classes to replace them.

Group 2: To be eligible for Group 2 you would need to have completed at least two full years of full-time, largely science based university education, including classes equivalent to the 4 Massey University veterinary prerequisite classes.

Massey University Class: Usual classes needed for credit

123.101 Chemistry and Living Systems: General chemistry + 1 sem. Organic chemistry

124.111 Physics for Life Sciences: 1 year of physics

162.101 Biology of Cells: (molecular) biology + First year biology series

199.101 Biology of Animals: Animal biology / vertebrate zoology + First year biology series

Each of the above classes should include laboratories and should be completed by the end of the fall semester in the year prior to matriculation (e.g., fall 2018 for matriculation in 2019).

Required undergraduate GPA

Group 1: Not applicable; courses completed in New Zealand.

Group 2: A minimum science GPA of 3.00 is required to be eligible for selection into the professional phase (Semester 2) of veterinary degree.

ADDITIONAL REQUIREMENTS AND CONSIDERATIONS

All VMCAS applicants must complete the supplemental application for Massey University. Your application will not be considered until you have submitted your online supplemental application.

The supplemental application consists of:
- An online Massey University application form for admission as an international student.

We also require the following but you usually do not need to supply these as they are sourced directly from NAVLE once you have completed your supplemental application:
- Your transcripts – from NAVLE application.
- Verification of your veterinary practical work experience – A letter signed by a veterinarian verifying you have completed a minimum of 10 days (80 hours) work experience at their clinic. ELoR's submitted by veterinarians as part of the VMCAS application can be substituted for the signed letter. Letters of recommendation are not required.

A bachelor's degree is not a prerequisite requirement for admission into the professional phase of the veterinary degree.

Is a Bachelor's Degree Required? no

Is this an International School? yes

ESTIMATED TUITION

Estimated Tuition Resident: Subsidized

Estimated Tuition Contract: 0

Estimated Tuition Non-Resident: $NZ 62,180 NZD per semester

AVAILABLE SEATS

Resident: 100

Contract: 0

Non-Resident: 24

VMCAS Participation: partial

Accepts International Students? yes

ADDITIONAL INFORMATION

Please note: The tuition fees are in New Zealand dollars. The actual cost in your currency will depend on the exchange rate at the time of paying tuition fees. The NZD is traditionally lower than the USD and CAD. Historically once conversion rates are accounted for, tuition fees at Massey University are usually in the third least expensive for out-of-state schools.

Application Deadline: 11/1/2018

VMCAS Deadline: 9/17/2018

UNIVERSITY OF MELBOURNE

Website: www.fvas.unimelb.edu.au

THE UNIVERSITY OF

MELBOURNE

SCHOOL DESCRIPTION

The University of Melbourne has a 150-year history of leadership in research, innovation, teaching and learning. Throughout its history the University of Melbourne has educated some of the world's most eminent scientists and researchers and this tradition continues today. Currently, we are the top ranked university in Australia.

The Melbourne Veterinary School's heritage began in 1886 as the first veterinary college in Australia, and we celebrated our centenary as a Faculty of the University of Melbourne in 2009. In July 2014, through consolidation of university faculties, the new Faculty of Veterinary and Agricultural Sciences was created. The Faculty is now comprised of the Melbourne Veterinary School and the School of Agriculture and Food. Our internationally accredited DVM degree program and our globally respected research and research-training programs are now taught and managed within The Melbourne Veterinary School.

> The University of Melbourne has a 150-year history of leadership in research, innovation, teaching and learning.

Our veterinary program is delivered across two sites: the city-center Parkville campus and the regional Werribee campus with our clinical teaching facilities. Our veterinary teaching hospital is designed to support top-class veterinary education with modern diagnostic capabilities including endoscopy, CT, MRI, image intensification, scintigraphy, on-site diagnostic pathology laboratories and a 24-hour small animal emergency and critical care unit. The university is currently transforming both campuses by constructing major additions to the veterinary teaching hospital and new state-of-the-art teaching facilities.

The veterinary program provides hands-on experience which includes industry integrated practical learning and clinical externship opportunities. Students gain experience in animal handling, care, and management by undertaking professional work-experience during and between the academic years. The school has strong programs in specialty disciplines for companion animals, horses, dairy cattle, sheep, and beef cattle. The school also has very strong primary care and emergency practices wherein DVM students gain Day-1 readiness. In addition to their broad-based core training, our students select a track in the third year to supplement their learning in a chosen area of interest. The tracks available are:

1. Production Animals
2. Small Animals
3. Horses
4. Government, Industry, and Conservation Health

Our DVM degree is accredited by the American Veterinary Medical Association (AVMA), by the Royal College of Veterinary Surgeons (UK), and by the Australasian Veterinary Boards Council Inc. These accreditations reflect the high quality and international standing of the course and permits graduates of the course to work as veterinarians in a wide range of countries including North America. Our success has been achieved by insisting on international excellence. Talented people from all over the world come to visit, study and work at the University of Melbourne. At last count, the University's student community of 44,000 included more than 9,800 international students from over 100 countries.

We invite you to join our tradition and discover why staff and students of the highest caliber are attracted to study at the Melbourne Veterinary School.

COURSE DURATION, ENTRY ROUTES AND STUDENT NUMBERS

The Melbourne Veterinary School offers studies in veterinary education through our professional entry graduate degree: the Doctor of Veterinary Medicine. The four-year degree offers veterinary students the best possible preparation for twenty-first century careers in a rapidly changing and increasingly global workforce. Students can enter the veterinary science program by one of two pathways:

1. As a graduate student by completing a science or agricultural science degree at another institution. Students who follow this pathway will enter the four-year graduate entry DVM program.

or at the University of Melbourne.

2. Via the undergraduate pathway by gaining entry to the Bachelor of Science degree at the University of Melbourne and achieving selection at the end of their second year.

NUMBER OF INTERNATIONAL STUDENTS THAT WE ACCEPT

Each year level has a total of 130 students with approximately 50 places reserved for international students.

PREREQUISITES FOR ADMISSION

1. Entrance to the DVM via the Melbourne Bachelor of Science: North American students should refer to the University's international prospectus for up to date details about entrance requirements for the Bachelor of Science by visiting www.coursesearch.unimelb.edu.au.

2. Entrance to the DVM as a graduate: Applicants will require a science or agricultural science degree from the University of Melbourne or another institution. Examples of appropriate degrees include Bachelor's degrees with majors in: Agriculture, Animal Science, Biochemistry, Biomedicine, Physiology or Zoology. Prerequisites for entry as a graduate are at least one semester of study in each of general or cellular biology and biochemistry as part of a science or agricultural degree.

3. Entrance to the DVM as an undergraduate: After completing prerequisite first and second year subjects in the Bachelor of Science, students will be eligible to apply for entry to the Veterinary Bioscience specialization of the Animal Health and Disease major in third year. Students who successfully complete their studies will have guaranteed entry into the DVM, with credit for one year of study, leaving three years of study in the DVM.

4. There is no standardized test or interview required.

APPLICATION INFORMATION

Students apply via VMCAS or via the International Admissions Office at the University of Melbourne. They can choose to apply online or apply through one of our overseas representatives. Visit https://futurestudents.unimelb.edu.au/info/international.

International applications via the International Admissions Office will be accepted throughout the year. Applications close in late December, for enrollment commencing in February the following year. Applicants are advised to apply as soon as possible to avoid disappointment. Applications will be considered as soon as they are received. We recognize the amount of time required by successful applicants to make arrangements for international travel and study and we attempt to give them as much advance notice as possible.

TUITION FEES

For information about tuition fees please visit:
- Undergraduate (e.g., Bachelor of Science) http://futurestudents.unimelb.edu.au/admissions/fees/ug-intl
- Graduate (e.g., DVM) http://futurestudents.unimelb.edu.au/admissions/fees/grad-intl

Application fee: AUD$100 (for applications via the International Admissions Office at the University of Melbourne)

Visas: All non-Australian students require a student visa, which is easily obtained following an offer of admission into our program. More information can be viewed on the website: www.services.unimelb.edu.au/international/visas/apply.

Deferments: Please note that successful applicants may not defer commencement of the DVM. Students can reapply for a start year intake when they are able to commence studies, and the application fee will be waived for international students.

NATIONAL AUTONOMOUS UNIVERSITY OF MEXICO (UNAM) COLLEGE OF VETERINARY MEDICINE

Email: lazq@unam.mx
Website: www.fmvz.unam.mx
escolar.fmvz.unam.mx

APPLICATION INFORMATION

Undergraduate admission of new students to the National Autonomous University of Mexico (UNAM) is done through the General Administration Scholar Affairs Direction (DGAE).

Students coming from high schools other than UNAM's own high school system compete for available places through a standardized test administered by UNAM. The test evaluates general abilities and knowledge in all areas, with emphasis on chemistry, biology, mathematics, and Spanish. Students taking the test are assigned to the Veterinary School according to the grade obtained (highest first), until the quota reserved for non-UNAM students is filled.

There are two annual applications dates: January and April. Information for specific applications dates can be reviewed at www.escolar .unam.mx (the semester starts in August).

In 2017, a total of 3,281 students applied for 85 places; the score of the accepted students in the standardized test was at least 108 out of 128 points.

> In 2017, a total of 3,281 students applied to UNAM for 85 places.

RESIDENCY IMPLICATIONS

There is no distinction between resident or nonresident students since UNAM is a Federal (National) University. Foreign students can also take the test and compete for the same pool of places, with the only extra requirement to pass a Spanish language test if their native language is not Spanish.

PREREQUISITES FOR ADMISSION

In order to be considered for admission, the students should have studied the secondary school and the high school at institutions with programs that are at least 75% equivalent to those of UNAM's own high school system, as evaluated by a revalidation committee. Thus, before being considered for admission, a student that completed high school in a foreign country should go through the revalidation process described here: http://www.dgire.unam.mx.

The committee will decide if, before being considered for admission, a prospective student has to pass examinations related to the courses lacking during his or her secondary and high school studies. Subjects reviewed include: mathematics (algebra, probability, statistics, trigonometry, geometry, differential and integral calculus); biological sciences (general biology, ecology, cell biology, anatomy, physiology, nutrition and metabolism, evolution, health education); chemistry (inorganic chemistry, organic chemistry, biochemistry). physics (general physics, thermodynamics, mechanics, electromagnetism, optics, acoustics, hydraulics); geography; history; and literature.

Required undergraduate GPA: It is not necessary

AP credit policy: Is not part of the admission requirements

Course completion deadline: It is based on the application dates, in January and June.

Standardized Examinations: As described before, admissions are based on a standardized test administered by UNAM.

Additional requirements and considerations: Foreign students must have a good command of the Spanish language

SUMMARY OF ADMISSION PROCEDURE

Timetable

Application dates can be checked at www.escolar .unam.mx

Deposit: It is not necessary

Deferments: Considered on an individual basis, and ordinarily granted for personal reasons, illness, lack of economic resources or other situations beyond the control of the students.

Evaluation criteria: Competition for available places through a standardized test administered by UNAM.

2017–2018 ADMISSIONS SUMMARY

Number of Applicants	Number of New Entrants
3,281	85 (2.6%)

EXPENSES FOR THE 2017–2018 ACADEMIC YEAR

(subject to change)

Tuition and fees: $500 USD per year

VETERINARIAN PROFILE: GAEMIA TRACY

YEAR OF GRADUATION
2012

PLACE OF EMPLOYMENT
Northstar VETS

What is your favorite aspect of being a veterinarian?
The thing I love most about my job is the daily opportunity to make a positive difference in pets' and pet owners' lives. With medical and surgical management of neurologic diseases, I am able to contribute to healing disease and improving the quality of life of the pets and their owners. The foundation for these skills were laid in veterinary school at The Ohio State University.

What type of veterinary medicine do you practice?
Veterinary neurology.

Where did you attend veterinary school?
The Ohio State University.

How long have you been practicing as a veterinarian?
Five years.

What advice do you have for those considering a career in veterinary medicine?
This must be something that you are passionate about—a good veterinarian never loses the desire to grow, develop, and sharpen his craft.

What challenges have you faced while practicing veterinary medicine?
There are always new and challenging procedures to perform, but the thing that has challenged me the most is maintaining a work-life balance. As a husband and a new father, it is important that I do well in all aspects of life and remain healthy. This requires 100% focus on the task at hand, whether it be providing medical care to a patient or crawling around with your children on the floor. I am also working on being thankful for every moment God provides for us in life, no matter how hard or difficult it may seem.

UNIVERSITÉ DE MONTRÉAL

Email: saefmv@medvet.umontreal.ca

Website: fmv.umontreal.ca/fmv

Université
de Montréal

APPLICATION INFORMATION

Applications available: November 1
    Online: 96,50$CAN

Application deadline: January 15

Residency implications: Canadian citizenship or permanent residency in Canada is required.

A total of 96 students are admitted each year.

> A total of 96 students are admitted each year. All lectures are given in French. Examinations must be written in French.

To be considered for admission, one must: a) meet the above requirements for citizenship, and b) have completed the required studies.

Note: All lectures are given in French. Examinations must be written in French.

The DMV is a 5-year program.

Condition concerning the knowledge of French: To be admissible, the candidate must demonstrate that he/she has acquired the minimal level of proficiency in French as required by the chosen program, as established by the University. To this end, the candidate must either:

- succeed the Épreuve uniforme de langue et littérature française of the Ministry of Education of Quebec or;
- obtain a score of at least 785/990 on the International French exam (Test de français international TFI).

Performance Score: This score is obtained by comparing the student's grade in each course with the class average.

Course completion deadline: The applicant must have completed all prerequisites at the time of application.

Additional considerations (in order of importance)
1. Academic record
2. Admission test

SUMMARY OF ADMISSION PROCEDURE

Timetable

Application deadline: January 15

Admission test: beginning of January to beginning of April (online test)

Notification of acceptance: mid-May

Fall semester begins: end of August

Deposit (to hold place in class): 300$CAN

Evaluation criteria	%
Performance score	60
Admission test	40

ESTIMATED EXPENSES FOR THE 2018–2019 ACADEMIC YEAR

Tuition and fees: 100$CAN per credit for residents of Quebec (approx. 45 per year)

300$CAN per credit for Canadian non-residents of Quebec

PREREQUISITES FOR ADMISSION

DEC (Diplôme d'Etudes Collégiales) including the following courses:

Course requirements

Physics   101, 201, 301–78

Chemistry   101, 201, 202

Biology   301, 401

Mathematics (including calculus)   103, 203

MURDOCH UNIVERSITY*

Email Address: international@murdoch.edu.au
Website: http://www.murdoch.edu.au/School-of-Veterinary-and
-Life-Sciences

SCHOOL DESCRIPTION

Western Australia is a beautiful part of Australia with a warm sunny climate. It has some of the world's most precious natural phenomena including Ningaloo Reef and the 350-million-year-old Bungle Bungle Range in the north, and the towering Karri forests of the south west. Perth is a modern, safe cosmopolitan city with a relaxed lifestyle that focuses on the outdoors. There are wineries, beaches, bushland, and unique wildlife within easy reach of the city, and a cosmopolitan mix of cafes, restaurants, pubs and thriving nightlife in the city center.

> Veterinary students learn in a true practice atmosphere with the final year of study devoted entirely to clinical exposure.

Murdoch University is a public university based in Perth, with campuses also in Singapore and Dubai. It began operations as the state's second university in 1973, and accepted its first students in 1975. The University is located 15km south of the central business district of Perth, and about 8 kilometers east of the port city of Fremantle. It currently is home to over 22,500 students including approximately 3,000 international students from over 90 countries.

Veterinary students from Murdoch graduate with a double degree (Bachelor of Science [Veterinary Biology] and Doctor of Veterinary Medicine) from a course that takes a total of five years to complete. The course is designed to enable students to acquire the knowledge and skills necessary for the diagnosis, treatment and prevention of disease in pets, farm animals, wildlife and laboratory animals. Veterinary students learn in a practice atmosphere with the final year of study lecture-free and devoted entirely to clinical exposure, including time spent at Perth Zoo.

The Veterinary Biology degree (3 years) encompasses both normal and abnormal aspects of vertebrate structure and function. The first year comprises units which introduce the scientific process, analysis of data and the form and function of the animal body; units in the second year include information on animal development, structure, function and metabolism; and units in the third year cover general aspects of the causes and nature of disease and its control. A further 6 trimesters of study over 2 calendar years leads to a Masters level degree of Doctor of Veterinary Medicine (DVM) which is a registrable veterinary qualification.

Murdoch students have access to excellent facilities, all on the one campus, including a 24-hour emergency clinic, large and small animal practices, an on campus farm and an equine hospital, as well as production animal and equine ambulatory services. The thriving practices have busy caseloads, serviced by many specialist clinicians, so that students can gain extensive experience.

The new BSc/DVM curriculum is designed to keep Murdoch at the forefront of veterinary education. This curriculum allows more time for students to develop areas of special interest through non-core rotations, externships and extramural experience. A Veterinary Professional Life stream is integrated throughout the course to assist students in their transition to future careers in veterinary science and provides a strong focus for developing professional life skills within the veterinary profession.

The veterinary science degree is accredited by the American Veterinary Medical Association (AVMA), the Royal College of Veterinary Surgeons (UK), and the Australian Veterinary Boards Council. Completing your Veterinary Science degree Murdoch saves you years of study, and potentially thousands of dollars; this is because with the correct preparation, the 4 years of veterinary specific tuition can be entered into after only one year of tertiary study in general biological science. Once you have finished your degree at Murdoch, you are eligible to sit your exams with the AVMA just as you would if you completed your studies in North America.

APPLICATION INFORMATION

For specific information (availability, deadlines, fees, and VMCAS participation), please refer to the contact information listed above.

All non-residents require a student visa, which is easily obtained following an offer of admission into the veterinary course. Applicants whose first language is not English must demonstrate competency in the English language, further details can be found at http://www.murdoch.edu.au/Future-students/International-students/Applying-to-Murdoch/English-requirements.

SUMMARY OF ADMISSIONS PROCEDURES

Timetable

There are four application deadlines each year, which are: March 31, June 30, September 30 and November 30.

School begins: mid-February

Some candidates may be eligible to begin in late July.

VMCAS application deadline: not applicable. Students are to apply direct via Murdoch. Application form can be found at http://www.murdoch.edu.au/Future-students/International-students/Applying-to-Murdoch/Application-forms

Deposit to hold a position: $1,000 AUD payable upon acceptance of offer

ENTRANCE REQUIREMENTS

Students who have completed one or more years of tertiary study and who have satisfied the appropriate prerequisites are eligible to apply for entry into second year of the 5-year program. Currently the prerequisites include units in chemistry, statistics and data analysis, introductory animal anatomy and physiology, cell and molecular biology and vertebrae structure and function, plus a unit that explores the basic building blocks for science students and another that introduces the history and philosophy of science and the interconnected nature of scientific disciplines. A unit covering the prin-

ciples of livestock science in an Australian context is also a prerequisite. This unit incorporates mandatory components that include animal handling competence of the common farm animals and a farm safety course. For students entering at the start of 2nd year a summer version of this unit is available.

Applications are also accepted from school leavers, with high achievers offered a place in the first year at Murdoch with a guaranteed progression into the veterinary specific course, provided they pass all first year units at the first attempt. Other applicants will be formally selected from those who have successfully completed one year or more of tertiary study, including the prerequisite units listed above, or equivalent units (excluding the livestock science unit). Applicants are required to supply with the application form (1) a curriculum vitae (CV) and (2) a typed Personal Statement of up to 500 words to which should be attached documents such references, and which should outline why you wish to become a veterinarian. You should include information such as how you consider your past study and experience to date will assist you to succeed in the veterinary course and in the veterinary profession. If you have any fails/late withdrawals in your post-secondary/tertiary study, you should explain the circumstances for your poor performance and why those circumstances will not apply to your Murdoch studies. You should aim to demonstrate your motivation and preparation for veterinary science

Assessment of the application will be based on the academic standard achieved in all previous tertiary study, the personal statement, and documented evidence of recent veterinary and animal related experience. Applicants who have satisfied the appropriate prerequisites may be offered a place in the second year of the BSc/DVM course. If not, an offer may be made into the first year of the course, with an assured progression into the second year after successful completion of all units in that year at the first attempt.

Deferments: considered on merit

Is a Bachelor's Degree Required? no

Is this an International School? yes

ESTIMATED TUITION

Estimated Tuition Resident: n/a

Estimated Tuition Contract: 0

Estimated Tuition Non-Resident: *A$29,000 progressing to *A$81,000 pa. *Based on 2015 values.

AVAILABLE SEATS

Resident: 0

Contract: 0

Non-Resident: 45

VMCAS Participation: non-VMCAS

Accepts International Students? yes

ADDITIONAL INFORMATION

Application Deadline: 11/20/2017

THE UNIVERSITY OF QUEENSLAND

Email Address: enquire@science.uq.edu.au
Website: veterinary-science.uq.edu.au

SCHOOL DESCRIPTION

The veterinary qualification of The University of Queensland (UQ) is accredited with the American Veterinary Medical Association, the Australasian Veterinary Boards Council (Australia and New Zealand), the Royal College of Veterinary Surgeons (United Kingdom), Malaysian Veterinary Council and the South African Veterinary Council.

The School of Veterinary Science's purpose-built facilities are located at UQ's Gatton campus and include Veterinary Teaching Laboratories, the Clinical Studies Centre, and the Veterinary Medical Centre (VMC) with fully equipped Equine and Companion Animal Hospitals, complete with the latest instrumentation for diagnostic imaging and surgical techniques. The VMC has recently commenced an ambulatory service for treatment of production animals on the rural properties surrounding the campus.

> The School has been recognised for a sustained record of excellence in teaching and learning.

The UQ Gatton campus is approximately 40 miles west of Brisbane, the capital city of the state of Queensland in Australia. The campus is easily accessible within one to two hours' drive from the major urban and tourism centres of Brisbane, the Gold Coast and Toowoomba, and has a rural atmosphere with on-campus access to domesticated animals including horses, cattle, pigs, poultry, cats, dogs and wildlife including kangaroos, reptiles and birds.

The School's co-location with the Queensland Animal Science Precinct makes the Gatton campus the most comprehensive animal research and training centre in Australia.

Since its first intake of students in 1936, the UQ School of Veterinary Science has been recognised for a sustained record of excellence in teaching and learning across the veterinary disciplines, and for the quality of its research.

With state-of-the-art facilities, and an ambitious academic recruitment program that has attracted an excellent cohort of staff, the School is at the forefront of veterinary education, supporting UQ's global ranking in the top 100 universities.

The diverse group of academic and clinical staff in the School, including those who have been recognised through nationally accredited awards, have made major contributions to tropical/subtropical animal health and medicine to benefit farm and companion animals, their owners and industry sectors.

The curriculum of the School of Veterinary Sciences is a 10-semester (5-year) program that runs from February to November in the first four years and November to October in the final year. The first year provides core foundational training in biological sciences, with emphases on animal biology, biochemistry, cellular physiology, anatomy and professional studies. In the second and third years, the emphasis becomes the understanding of diseases, and their causation, diagnosis, treatment and prevention. In the fourth year, a strong clinical focus is provided, which is then reinforced in fifth year through 38 weeks of core and elective clinical rotations, both in the Veterinary Medical Centre and off-campus practices.

A strong commitment to research training in veterinary sciences is provided through clinical research electives. The School of Veterinary Science has outstanding teaching and research programs encompassing all aspects of veterinary science, with particular strengths in biosecurity and infectious diseases, genetics, medicine, nutrition, Australian wildlife, farm animal and equine medicine, production and reproduction.

APPLICATION INFORMATION

For specific information on applying for a place in the program, please refer to the UQ Science Prospectus, which is updated annually (science.uq.edu.au/prospectus).

The school enrols approximately 120-130 students annually, of which up to 40 seats are held for international students. International students must hold a student visa for the duration of their studies.

SUMMARY OF ADMISSIONS PROCEDURES

There are no specific interviews for international applicants. From 2019 onwards, non-resident applicants may be required to successfully complete an online situational judgement test as an admission requirement.

International applicants for the program at UQ can submit an application directly to the university or through one of UQ's authorised International Education Representatives (future-students.uq.edu.au/find-international-representative)

Domestic students, or international students studying in Australia, may apply for entry through the Queensland Tertiary Admissions Centre (qtac.edu.au).

Successful applicants can apply to defer for one year after receiving an offer of a seat in the program.

Is a Bachelor's Degree Required? no

Is this an International School? yes

ESTIMATED TUITION

Information about fees for international students can be found on The University of Queensland Future Students website (future-students.uq.edu.au/apply/undergraduate/international/fees). Fees are subject to annual indexation (ppl.app.uq.edu.au/content/9.30.02-student-fees-and-charges).

Information about fees for domestic students can be found on The University of Queensland Future Students website (future-students.uq.edu.au/apply/undergraduate/fees). Fees are subject to annual indexation (ppl.app.uq.edu.au/content/9.30.02-student-fees-and-charges).

Full-time enrolment consists of 16 units per annum or 80 units for the veterinary science program.

AVAILABLE SEATS

Domestic: 80

International: 40

VMCAS Participation: non-VMCAS

Accepts International Students? yes

APPLICATION DEADLINE

International applicants are eligible to participate in streamlined visa processing. It is recommended that international student applications are received by UQ by 30 November in the year preceding entry.

CRICOS Provider Number 00025B

ROSS UNIVERSITY SCHOOL OF VETERINARY MEDICINE

Email Address: VetAdmissions@RossU.edu
Website: veterinary.rossu.edu

ROSS UNIVERSITY
SCHOOL OF VETERINARY MEDICINE

SCHOOL DESCRIPTION

Ross University School of Veterinary Medicine (Ross Vet), located in St. Kitts, West Indies, offers an accredited DVM program focused on educating tomorrow's leaders and discoverers in veterinary medicine. Ross Vet holds current accreditation from the American Veterinary Medical Association (AVMA*) and the St. Kitts and Nevis Accreditation Board. At Ross Vet, our passion is training students to become the next generation of career-ready, compassionate veterinarians. Our 4,000+ graduates are successfully practicing veterinary medicine across the US, Canada, and beyond.

> Discover a world of possibilities in veterinary medicine at Ross Vet.

The seven-semester pre-clinical curriculum is enhanced by hands-on clinical experience to help prepare students for the final year of clinical training at one of Ross Vet's affiliated AVMA-accredited schools in the US, UK, Canada, Australia, New Zealand, and Ireland. Ross Vet's faculty have outstanding credentials in teaching and research and share a passion for educating the veterinarians of tomorrow. Ross Vet operates on a three-semester per year calendar.

Each semester is 15 full academic weeks, including final exams. Ross Vet graduates are eligible to practice veterinary medicine in all 50 states, Canada and Puerto Rico upon completion of the requisite licensing requirements. Ross Vet students who are U.S. citizens/permanent residents and meet the Department of Education's qualifying criteria may be eligible for Federal Stafford Loans and Federal Graduate PLUS Loans.

APPLICATION INFORMATION

- Students can apply through VMCAS or directly through Ross Vet.

EVALUATION CRITERIA

- Undergraduate cumulative grade point average (GPA)

- GPA in required pre-veterinary coursework

- Advanced science courses (Cell Biology, Genetics, Microbiology, Anatomy and Physiology, etc.)

- Graduate Record Examination (GRE) scores

- Personal essay

- Letters of recommendation from academic and/or professional references (at least one letter should be from a veterinarian)

- Extracurricular activities and accomplishments

- Personal qualities

- Personal interview

- Record of professional veterinary experience (working with animals or veterinary research) - at least 150 hours

SUMMARY OF ADMISSIONS PROCEDURES

Timetable (for VMCAS applications)

Application deadline: September 17, 2018 at 12 Midnight Eastern Time

Date interviews are held: Year-round

Date acceptances mailed: As soon as possible after the interview

School begins: Three start dates per year: September, January and May

TIMETABLE

Application deadline: None; rolling admissions

Date interviews are held: Year-round

Date acceptances mailed: As soon as possible after the interview

School begins: Three start dates per year: September, January and May

Deposit (to hold place in class): $1,000.00

Deferments: Considered

ENTRANCE REQUIREMENTS

To be considered for review by the admission committee the applicant must complete at least 48 credits of college work.

Course completion deadline: Required courses must be completed prior to enrollment.

AP credit policy: Must appear on official college transcripts.

Standardized Examinations: Results of the Graduate Record Examination (GRE) are required.

Is a Bachelor's Degree Required? no

Is this an International School? yes

ESTIMATED TUITION

Resident and Non-Resident: $18,310**

AVAILABLE SEATS

Resident and Non-Resident: 130

TEST REQUIREMENTS

Results of the Graduate Record Examination (GRE) are required.

English Language Proficiency: Applicants presenting fewer than 60 upper division credits from an English language college or university must provide the official record of the scores for the Test of English as a Foreign Language (TOEFL). The Admissions Committee prefers to see an overall score of 100 or better on the TOEFL.

VMCAS Participation: partial

Accepts International Students? yes

ADDITIONAL INFORMATION

Application Deadline: 9/17/2018

---

* Ross Vet's Doctor of Veterinary Medicine degree is accredited by the AVMA COE. AVMA Council on Education.
Phone: 800-248-2862 www.avma.org

**Tuition rates are subject to change

ROYAL VETERINARY COLLEGE

Email Address: admissions@rvc.ac.uk
Website: www.rvc.ac.uk

SCHOOL DESCRIPTION

Founded in 1791, the Royal Veterinary College (RVC), University of London, is at the forefront of teaching, research, and practice in biological sciences and veterinary medicine, and has been behind some important advances in the history of disease control, evolution, and human and animal welfare and medicine.

We are an international institution, with a worldwide reputation. Our students come from 54 countries, and our staff from 95 countries. We have a successful record of training North American students and can count several hundred American and Canadian graduates as alumni.

RVC lecturers are experts and active researchers in their field, and the College offers exciting research opportunities, providing an unrivalled learning experience to take your knowledge to the highest level and to help shape the future of science.

The RVC has two campuses, one in London and one on the outskirts of London, in Hertfordshire.

Our London campus is in Camden, one of the most creative and stimulating areas of the city. Famous for its markets, vibrant culture, and music venues, Camden is an exciting place to experience student life. It is also home to a beautiful canal and lock, Regent's Park, ZSL London Zoo, and the iconic Roundhouse music venue.

> The Royal Veterinary College is at the forefront of teaching and research in veterinary medicine, veterinary nursing, and biological sciences.

Our historic Camden Campus is where veterinary medicine students will spend their first two years as well as first-year students of the Graduate Accelerated programme. Biosciences students study at the Camden Campus throughout their course.

You will also find on campus an anatomy museum, our first opinion animal hospital, and the London Bioscience and Innovation Centre, the home of over forty biotechnology and life sciences companies, from small start-ups to established, global players.

The Hawkshead Campus, Hertfordshire, is equipped with facilities tailored to deliver both the theoretical and practical elements of your course. It is where veterinary medicine students are based for the final three years of their course, alongside veterinary nursing students and specialists-in-training.

The self-contained Campus houses modern lecture theatres and laboratories, a large library, and a learning resource centre. There are also a number of specialist centres on campus, including the Centre for Emerging and Endemic Diseases, Structure and Motion Laboratory, Clinical Skills Centre, and Clinical Investigations Centre.

You will also find on campus the small animal referrals hospital, one of the largest and most advanced veterinary hospitals in the world treating over 9,000 cases each year, the equine hospital, and Boltons Park Farm, our farm animal teaching facility.

Places in RVC halls of residence are available and students from overseas are guaranteed a place if requested. The College has a number of dedicated staff who provide academic and pastoral support to students throughout the course, and we have an active and welcoming student community.

APPLICATION INFORMATION

For specific application information (availability, deadlines, fees and VMCAS participation), please refer to our website at https://www.rvc.ac.uk/study/northamerica.

Residency implications: The UK government introduced a points-based immigration system for students from non-EU countries who wish to study in the UK. For further information on entry to the UK, please refer to https://www.gov.uk/browse/visas-immigration/student-visas and to the College's web site. Students must also be able to ensure adequate financial support for the duration of their course.

SUMMARY OF ADMISSIONS PROCEDURES

Timetable

VMCAS application deadline: Monday, September 17, 2018 at 12 Midnight Eastern Time

Interview dates are arranged: October

Date interviews are held: November (Interviews for North American candidates normally take place in the USA.)

Date acceptances mailed: January to March

School begins: September

Transcripts: All transcripts to VMCAS by 17 September. But aim for 1 September in case of problems.

Deposit (to hold place in class): Offers are conditional of payment of a deposit and visa paperwork will not be issued until a deposit is paid. Amount will be advised at point of offer.

Deferments: may be considered in exceptional circumstances.

EVALUATION CRITERIA

Academic performance
Animal/veterinary experience
Interview
An academic reference must be provided. Reference(s) will also be required to demonstrate experience in animal and veterinary environments.
Personal statement

ENTRANCE REQUIREMENTS

Course requirements

VMCAS applicants are normally final year or recent university graduates although students with two years pre-vet will be considered. We will also consider High School students studying AP or the International Baccalaureate. These students apply through UCAS (see our website at https://www.rvc.ac.uk/study/northamerica). Science graduates or applicants in the final year of a science based degree with the prerequisites may be considered for our 4 year accelerated course. Applicants who are unsuccessful in gaining a place on the four year programme may be considered for our five year programme. Required at upper level (i.e., 300-400 level): At least 8 upper-level credits in Biology/Biological Science. Examples include but are not limited to: Animal Biology, Physiology, Anatomy, Zoology, Microbiology or Genetics.

Also required (4 semester credits each): Biochemistry, Physics, Mathematics, Anatomy/Physiology, Organic Chemistry, and Biology.

Required undergraduate GPA: 3.40 or higher preferred (on 4.0 point scale).

AP credit policy: not applicable for graduate applicants.

Course completion deadline: all required courses should be completed by July of the year of admissions.

Standardized examinations: GRE General test required and must be sent to the College by 15 September. RVC institution code is 3207.

ADDITIONAL REQUIREMENTS AND CONSIDERATIONS

Applicants are also expected to have gained at least 70 hours of experience in a veterinary setting and at least 70 hours of animal handling experience in the 18 months prior to application. The experience can be paid or voluntary and in any relevant environment outside of the applicant's home/personal setting.

Supplemental Application: see website

Is a Bachelor's Degree Required? no

Is this an International School? yes

ESTIMATED TUITION

Estimated Tuition Resident: pending, see our website for further information

Estimated Tuition Contract: none

Estimated Tuition Non-Resident: pending, see our website for further information

AVAILABLE SEATS

Resident: tbc

Contract: none

Non-Resident: tbc

TEST REQUIREMENTS

Standardized examinations: GRE General test required and to be submitted to the RVC by 17 September. RVC institution code is 3207.

VMCAS Participation: partial

Accepts International Students? yes

ADDITIONAL INFORMATION

Application Deadline: 9/17/2018

PRE-VETERINARY PROFILE: CAROLINE OTTO

Current School Name
Rowan University

What type of veterinary medicine are you interested in pursuing, and why?
I'm hoping to become a wildlife and conservation or zoo vet after veterinary school. I want to be able to help and give a voice to animals who aren't usually taken care of by most of society.

What is/was your major during undergraduate school?
I am a biological studies major at Rowan University. I am minoring in chemistry and psychology and have concentrations in neuroscience and honors studies.

What are your short-term and long-term goals?
My short-term goal for now is to get into vet school! I'm in the application process and it's been quite a year, but I'm finally close to reaching this goal. As for the long term, I want to work toward opening a veterinary school in New Jersey. Not having an in-state school made the decision to go to vet school really difficult for me, so I'm hoping to help other students in my position so they don't to worry about that.

What are you doing as an applicant/pre-vet to prepare for veterinary school?
The biggest thing I'm doing right now is working as a veterinary technician. This has given me some incredible insight into what daily life is like as a veterinarian and some of the challenges I will face. It has prepared me for what life might be like for me after graduation, and it has confirmed for me that this is truly what I want to do with my life. I've also been volunteering at a charity wildlife refuge for the past year and a half. It's been so fulfilling to get to rehabilitate wildlife and see them released back into the wild.

What extracurricular activities are you involved in currently?
Last year, I started a pre-vet club at Rowan University. I felt like we needed somewhere for pre-vet students to meet one another and help each other out. This year we've had several guest speakers, including some representatives from vet schools, and we have talked about the application process. Next semester, we're hoping to have our first field trip to Cornell's open house and hold mock interviews for students who are interested! I am also President of the Honors Book Group, something that is so much fun for me. I've met so many fun and amazing people who just want to talk about good books with me—it's been a great stress reliever.

How old were you when you first became interested in being a veterinarian?
I think I've always known deep down that I wanted to become a veterinarian or at least work with animals, but it took me a while to really commit to it and realize that the other interests I was pursuing weren't really making me happy. It wasn't until my sophomore year of college that I really committed myself to this path.

Please describe your various experiences in preparation for applying to veterinary school.
I've made spreadsheets to try to analyze what schools I had the best chance of attending, which ones I liked the most, and which might give me the most financial aid. I've completed mock interviews to prepare myself, and I've read everything I could find on how to make myself a stronger candidate. I've also tried to diversify my experience as much as possible to find out what I really want so I can communicate a real understanding of my future career goals during the application and interview process. Oh, and lots of deep breaths and tea!

What characteristics are you looking for in a veterinary school?
First and foremost, I want a school that is trying to foster veterinarians who use medicine to give back. Whether that's through a wildlife hospital, a shelter medicine program, or helping out the local community after a natural disaster, I want to know that my school is working to help people and animals. I also want a really strong sense of community. Veterinary school can and will be very stressful, so I want to feel like my peers and professors want me to succeed and are willing to help me—just like I want to help them.

What advice do you have for other pre-veterinary students?
Work hard! If you really commit to becoming a veterinarian and give it everything you have, there's no reason you can't do it, even if it's not until your third try. I've worked harder for this than I have for anything else in my life, and no matter how long it takes, I know I'm going to get there—and you will too!

UNIVERSITY OF SASKATCHEWAN
WESTERN COLLEGE OF VETERINARY MEDICINE

Email Address: wcvm.admissions@usask.ca

Website: www.usask.ca/wcvm

SCHOOL DESCRIPTION

The Western College of Veterinary Medicine is located in the city of Saskatoon, which has a population of about 265,000 and is the major urban center in central Saskatchewan. The city is also the major commercial center for central and northern Saskatchewan and is served by 2 national airlines with direct connections to all major centers in Canada.

The Western College of Veterinary Medicine is one of the few veterinary colleges where all health sciences and agriculture are offered on the same campus. The college is devoted to undergraduate education and has a reputation in Canada and in the northwestern United States for educating veterinarians who are well-rounded in general veterinary medicine and have good practical backgrounds. It has one of the best field-service caseloads in North America.

> The Western College of Veterinary Medicine has one of the best field-service caseloads in North America.

APPLICATION INFORMATION

For specific application information (availability, deadlines, fees, and VMCAS participation), please refer to the contact information listed above.

Residency implications: Currently, 78 students are selected for quota positions from Alberta, British Columbia, Manitoba, Saskatchewan, and the Yukon, Nunavut, and Northwest Territories. Special consideration is given to self identified individuals of aboriginal origin. Residents of foreign countries are not considered.

SUMMARY OF ADMISSIONS PROCEDURES

Timetable

Application deadline: December 1

Reference deadline: February 15

Date interviews are held: May–June

Date acceptances mailed: on or before July 1

School begins: late August

Deposit (to hold place in class): none required.

Deferments: not considered.

EVALUATION CRITERIA

The 3-part admission procedure consists of an assessment of academic ability, a personal interview, and an overall assessment of the application file.

% weight

Grades 60%

Interview* 40%

* Interview selection is based entirely on academic performance.

ENTRANCE REQUIREMENTS

Required undergraduate GPA: a minimum cumulative average of 75% is required.

Course completion deadline: prerequisite courses must be completed by the time of entry into the program.

Standardized examinations: none required.

PREREQUISITES FOR ADMISSION

Course Description	Number of Hours/Credits	Necessity
English	6	Required
Physics	3	Required
Biology	6	Required
Genetics	3	Required
Introductory Chemistry	6	Required
Organic Chemistry	3	Required
Mathematics or Statistics	6	Required
Biochemistry	3	Required
Microbiology	3	Required
Electives	21	Required

Reference Forms: Two required—one from a veterinarian and one from an individual with an agricultural- or animal-related background.

Additional Requirements/Information: Space is provided on the application form to nominate referees to support the application. Referees will be contacted directly and asked to complete the reference form online.

ADDITIONAL REQUIREMENTS AND CONSIDERATIONS

Animal/veterinary work experience, motivation, and knowledge

Maturity

Leadership

Communication skills

Is a Bachelor's Degree Required? no

Is this an International School? no

ESTIMATED TUITION

Estimated Tuition Resident: $$10,131

Estimated Tuition Contract: $$10,131

Estimated Tuition Non-Resident: $$10,131

AVAILABLE SEATS

Resident: 20

Contract: 57

Non-Resident: 1

TEST REQUIREMENTS

None

VMCAS Participation: non-VMCAS

Accepts International Students? no

ADDITIONAL INFORMATION

Application Deadline: 12/1/2018 for fall 2019 entry

ST. GEORGE'S UNIVERSITY

Email Address: SGUEnrolment@sgu.edu
Website: www.sgu.edu

St. George's University

SCHOOL DESCRIPTION

Having received full accreditation by the AVMA COE in 2011, St. George's University School of Veterinary Medicine is proud of its academic excellence exemplified by its breadth of highly regarded education, unprecedented student support services, and internationally recognized faculty. The core mission of the University is creating excellent academic programs within an international setting where students and faculty are actively recruited from around the world. St. Georges University has drawn faculty and students from over 140 countries, assembling a diverse community of disparate cultural and educational backgrounds.

> SGU prepares its students for leadership, life-long success and service in a constantly changing world.

Located on the southwest corner of the Caribbean island of Grenada, St. George's shoreline location offers its growing student body a serene environment in which to live, learn and create a worldwide network of friends and colleagues. Along with St. George's state-of-the-art facilities, complete with a large animal facility and, marine station, and the SGU Small Animal Clinic, St. George's University School of Veterinary Medicine prepares its students for leadership, life-long success and service in a constantly changing world.

Over 6,000 students from throughout the world are enrolled in the University's School of Medicine, School of Veterinary Medicine, School of Arts and Sciences or graduate programs which include a CEPH-accredited MPH and MBA program. SGU students also benefit from world-renowned international academic partnerships with universities, hospitals and other educational and scientific institutions.

The veterinary medical program is delivered with a number of entry options: the seven-, six- and five-year programs which begin with the preveterinary medical sciences and an option to enter directly into the four-year veterinary medical program. This enables students flexible entry points depending upon their academic backgrounds. Students accepted into the preveterinary medical sciences are placed in the appropriate program option (either the seven-, six- or five-year program track) according to their academic background and are enrolled in the veterinary medical program for five to seven years. Applicants accepted directly into the veterinary medical sciences generally complete the program in four years.

The DVM program is conducted on the University's main campus on the True Blue peninsula of Grenada, West Indies, except for the final year which is the clinical year spent at an affiliated AVMA-accredited School of Veterinary Medicine. These schools are located in the United States, Canada, United Kingdom, Ireland, and Australia.

APPLICATION INFORMATION

As a member of the Association of American Veterinary Medical Colleges (AAVMC) the School of Veterinary Medicine participates in the AAVMC's centralized Veterinary Medical College Application Service (VMCAS). Aspiring veterinary medical students have the option of applying to the January 2019 or August 2019 entering class through the VMCAS 2018 application cycle. Candidates who intend to apply to veterinary schools through VMCAS can include St. George's University as a designated school and

PREREQUISITES FOR ADMISSION		
Course Description	Number of Hours/Credits	Necessity
General Biology or Zoology with Lab	8	Required
Inorganic Chemistry (general or Physical) with lab	8	Required
Organic Chemistry with lab	4	Required
Biochemistry	3	Required
Genetics	3	Required
Physics with lab	4	Required
Calculus, Computer Science or Statistics	3	Required
English	3	Required

follow the instructions for the SGU supplemental application. To learn more or apply go to http://aavmc .org/Students-Applicants-and-Advisors.aspx.

If you are not applying through VMCAS we encourage you to apply online through the SGU website at www.sgu.edu/apply-now/index.html. As an alternative, you can still download a paper copy to print and complete manually.

SUMMARY OF ADMISSIONS PROCEDURES

Application Deadlines for August and January Matriculation: The Committee on Admission utilizes a rolling admission policy in the School of Veterinary Medicine; therefore, applications are accepted and reviewed on an ongoing basis. The final deadline for receipt of direct (non-VMCAS) applications and all supporting documentation is April 15 of the current year for the August class, and November 15 of the preceding year for the January class. Prospective candidates should note that the entering classes are highly competitive and those applications completed early have the advantage of being reviewed at the beginning of the admission process. The time necessary to secure official transcripts, standardized test scores, and letters of recommendation should be taken into consideration. The Committee reserves the right to defer an application to the following semester if there are no available seats.

The Office of Admission will acknowledge receipt of a candidate's application within two weeks of its arrival. A candidate will be informed of any required supporting documents missing at that time. Within one month after receipt of all application materials, a candidate will receive notice that the application is complete and being reviewed to determine whether an interview will be granted.

The Office of Admission encourages candidates who have been approved for an interview to request interviews in Grenada, and will schedule one upon the applicant's request. The University recognizes that financial considerations may prevent many candidates who reside at great distances from Grenada from choosing this option.

Interviews, therefore, may be conducted in the United States, the United Kingdom, Canada, the Caribbean, or other locations that best serve the diverse applicant pool. Candidates are advised that being granted an interview is no guarantee of acceptance; the interview itself plays a significant part in the decision by the Committee on Admission. Applicants are notified of the decision of the Committee on Admission. A record of the notification is kept for one year.

ENTRANCE REQUIREMENTS

The requirements for direct entry into the four-year DVM program vary depending on the educational system of your home country. What is required for all applicants is completion of secondary school, a period of farm experience or time spent in a veterinary practice, and possession of a bachelors degree from an accredited University or 60 credit hours.

Specific undergraduate coursework (or its equivalent) is required as part of the preveterinary medical sciences requirements for admission.

Two letters of recommendation. In order of importance to the Committee on Admission, these are the categories:

a. A veterinarian with whom you have worked

b. A university professor (or, for those applying for the preveterinary program, a teacher)

c. A preveterinary advisor committee, or an advisor/ counselor.

One essay: A personal statement discussing the significant factors which led to your decision to pursue a career in veterinary medicine, and how you see yourself using this career to make a difference in the world (maximum 1500 words).

Applicants from North America

A completed bachelors degree from an accredited university is required for direct entry into the four-year veterinary medical program. A candidate may apply before completion of the degree. Under exceptional circumstances a candidate may be considered with 60 undergraduate credit hours.

Standardized Examination: Candidates must submit scores by the corresponding application deadlines (see below) on the Graduate Record Examination or alternatively on the MCAT. (Our GRE Code is 7153; MCAT code 21303.)

Applicants from Other Systems of Education

For direct entry into the four-year DVM program, a bachelors degree with a strong science background is required.

Applicants with passes at the Advanced Level of the General Certificate of Education will be assessed individually and will be considered for appropriate entry into the five-year DVM program. Generally, A Level students with the appropriate courses and grades matriculate into the five-year veterinary medical program.

If English is not the principal language, the applicant must have achieved a score in the Test of English as a Foreign Language (TOEFL) of at least 600 points, 250 points computer-based or 100 points internet-based.

Is a Bachelor's Degree Required? yes

Is this an International School? yes

ESTIMATED TUITION

Estimated Tuition Resident/Sponsored: $37,898 per year

Estimated Tuition Contract: 0

Estimated Tuition Non-Resident/Non-Sponsored: $37,898 per year

AVAILABLE SEATS

Each class consists of 110 students. No preference is given to applicant's place of residence.

TEST REQUIREMENTS

Standardized Examination: Candidates must submit scores by the corresponding application deadlines (see below) on the Graduate Record Examination or alternatively on the MCAT. (If sending GRE Scores directly to SGU use School Code 7153. If sending GRE scores to VMCAS use School Code 7402.) For the most current GRE submission information, please see https://portal.vmcas.org/vmcasHelpPages/instructions/academic-history/tests/index.html.

VMCAS Participation: partial

Accepts International Students? yes

ADDITIONAL INFORMATION

Dual Degree Programs

Combined DVM/MPH, MSc, and MBA degree programs are available. Applications can be submitted online directly through the SGU website at www.sgu.edu or via the VMCAS application system. If you have questions about the application process, please call one of our admission advisors at 1 (800) 899-6337, ext 1280.

Application Deadline: 9/17/2018

SYDNEY SCHOOL OF VETERINARY SCIENCE

Email: vet.science@sydney.edu.au

Website: sydney.edu.au/vetscience

THE UNIVERSITY OF

SYDNEY

SCHOOL INFORMATION

As Australia's first university, the University of Sydney's reputation spans more than 160 years. We are regularly ranked in the top 0.3% of universities worldwide. We teach more than 60,000 bright minds, with over 10,000 international students from more than 145 countries. We've taught 145 Olympians, 6 prime ministers, 2 Nobel laureates, 3 astronauts, 110 Rhodes scholars and 1 Pulitzer Prize winner. When you come to study at the University of Sydney, you become part of an inspiring network of leading academics, and distinguished graduates and alumni.

> The University of Sydney's School of Veterinary Science delivers inspirational and innovative student-centered teaching

Located only ten minutes by bus from the heart of the Sydney business district, the main Camperdown campus provides easy access to Sydney's vibrant social scene, Sydney harbour and surrounds.

One of the best aspects of studying at the University of Sydney is that it is located in the most beautiful city in the 'down-under' country of Australia, which is a young, modern and dynamic city.

The Sydney School of Veterinary Science was established in 1910 and is the oldest continuing School of its kind in Australia. We are an international leader in veterinary and animal education and ranked as Australia's top university and equal 11th in the world for veterinary science in the latest QS World University Rankings (2017). We received a score of 5/5 from Excellence in Research for Australia (ERA) for veterinary science research. The School delivers inspirational and innovative student-centered teaching emphasizing life-long, evidence-based learning whilst also providing clinical and research excellence through creative, collaborative programs.

We maintain teaching hospitals on both the inner-city Camperdown campus and the rural Camden campus, where you will work with veterinarians in a clinical teaching and learning environment. Referral and primary accession cases are seen at both sites. The University Veterinary Teaching Hospital at Camden also provides veterinary services to farms in the region, while the Wildlife Health and Conservation Clinic provides veterinary services to sick and injured Australian native wildlife; reptiles; and avian, aquatic and exotic pets. A wide range of companion animals, farm animals, racing animals, exotic and native species are seen. We have a strong global network of more than 5,000 alumni across the veterinary, agricultural, and public health sectors, including graduates in North America and Canada. Our active student societies, including VetSoc and the Camden Farms Society, ensure a rich and rewarding experience both in and out of the classroom.

The Doctor of Veterinary Medicine (DVM) program aims to produce career ready graduates with excellent fundamental knowledge and skills in managing animal health and disease; and in protecting and advancing animal, human and environmental health and welfare locally and globally. Clinical exposure, clinical skills training and animal handling commence in the first semester and continue throughout the course. The program culminates in a lecture-free capstone experience year where you will be placed as an intern in a variety of different veterinary clinics and in a wide range of locations, including rotations in the University Teaching Hospitals at Sydney and Camden and in our Wildlife Health and Conservation Clinic.

The DVM program will equip you with the knowledge and skills to choose from many career options as a veterinary professional participating in the care and welfare of animals. Completion of the course will provide you with a wide knowledge of the principles associated with every aspect of health and disease in animals—domestic and wild.

ENTRY PATHWAYS

The University of Sydney has two pathways for you to study veterinary medicine:

1. *Undergraduate applicants:* You can apply for entry into a combined six-year Bachelor of Veterinary Biology/Doctor of Veterinary Medicine (BVetBiol/DVM) on the basis of your secondary school results (plus additional selection criteria). The BVetBiol/DVM commences with two years of undergraduate study in the Bachelor of Veterinary Biology and if you perform well you will be eligible to progress to the Doctor of Veterinary Medicine in years 3-6. Undergraduate applications must be direct to the University.

2. *Graduate applicants:* If you have completed a bachelor degree, and have completed the prerequisite subjects* you can apply for entry into the four-year DVM program. Graduate DVM applications are through VMCAS.

*Prerequisites for the DVM are the successful completion of at least one semester of study in general chemistry (physical and inorganic), organic chemistry, biology and biochemistry. University of Sydney units of study that meet the prerequisite requirements are provided as examples of the content that all applicants are assumed to have, these can be found on: http://sydney.edu.au/courses/doctor-of-veterinary-medicine

ADMISSION REQUIREMENTS

Academic Performance:
1. If you are applying as an undergraduate for the BVetBiol/DVM, you will be assessed on the basis of your academic achievement in your final year of secondary education (Year 12 or equivalent) or your tertiary stud-

ies from a recognized University. Minimum GPA required for BVetBiol/DVM entry is 2.80 on a 4.00 scale, and you must demonstrate an aptitude for science-based study.

2. If you are applying as a graduate for the DVM, you will be assessed on the basis of your completed bachelor degree from the University of Sydney or another accredited institution, along with your relevant work experience. Minimum GPA required for DVM entry is 2.80 on a 4.00 scale. You must have successfully completed the prerequisite subjects, which can be found on http://sydney.edu.au/vetscience/dvm/prerequisites.shtml.

3. *Additional requirements and considerations:* You are expected to have gained relevant work experience and animal handling. You must demonstrate your relevant work experience in your application. Please note, applicants applying for the graduate entry DVM through VMCAS do not need to complete the supplementary application form. For graduate entry, the minimum work experience is four weeks, undertaken within two years of the application date.

PRACTICAL EXPERIENCE

During the inter-semester and intra-semester breaks you will be required to undertake placements for preparatory clinical and animal husbandry experience. The final year is free of lectures, and instead, you will participate in practice-based activities and the management and care of patients.

PROFESSIONAL RECOGNITION

Sydney graduates are immediately eligible for registration for practice with the Veterinary Practitioners Board in each Australian state and territory and are recognised by the Royal College of Veterinary Surgeons in the United Kingdom and the American Veterinary Medical Association.

APPLICATION INFORMATION

As an international student, you can apply directly to the University of Sydney using the on-line application: http://sydney.edu.au/courses. In addition, for the DVM you are able to apply through VMCAS.

You may also be interested in obtaining information about the University of Sydney from one of these University representatives: https://sydney.edu.au/future-students/international/undergraduate/find-an-agent.php

VMCAS application deadline: Monday, September 17, 2018 at 12 Midnight Eastern Time

Direct Application Deadline: Applicants need to check the website for the 2018 opening and closing dates: https://sydney.edu.au/vetscience/dvm/entry.shtml. It should be noted the semester for the four-year DVM program commences in early February each year.

Application dates and details can be found on the future student website at https://sydney.edu.au/future-students or http://sydney.edu.au/vetscience/dvm/entry.shtml

NEW ENTRANTS

Bachelor of Veterinary Biology/DVM:

Australian Resident: 40

International: 40

Doctor of Veterinary Medicine (Graduate entry):

Australian Resident: 30

International: 30

TUITION FEES 2019 (INDICATIVE FEES)

Information on tuition fees can be found on the website relating to each degree:

http://sydney.edu.au/courses/bachelor-of-veterinary-biology-and-doctor-of-veterinary-medicine

http://sydney.edu.au/courses/doctor-of-veterinary-medicine

UTRECHT UNIVERSITY

Email: BIC00902@uu.nl

Website: www.uu.nl/en/education/veterinary-education

SHORT HISTORY

In 1821 a state veterinary school was founded in Utrecht. Almost a century later, in 1918, the school acquired the status of an institution of higher learning and in 1925 it was incorporated into the State University of Utrecht and thereby became the first and until to date the only Faculty of Veterinary Medicine in the Netherlands. Utrecht University, founded in 1636, is one of the 14 universities in the Netherlands. The faculty of Veterinary Medicine is now one of the 6 faculties of Utrecht University and is located at campus site De Uithof just outside the city of Utrecht. The Faculty of Veterinary Medicine is housed in modern and spacious buildings on a total surface of 60.000 m.

> Utrecht University is one of the 14 universities in the Netherlands and is located at campus site De Uithof.

ORGANISATION AND STAFF

The faculty encompasses 8 departments with specialized facilities, a Faculty Office and a number of general services (e.g. leaning environment with audio-visual units and the library, pharmacy, experimental farms, museum, student computer rooms etc). Most staff members can communicate well in English and most lecturers have experience in teaching veterinary medicine in the English language.

VETERINARY EDUCATION

Admission of students to the 6-year veterinary training programme (taught in Dutch) is limited to 225 each year, resulting in a total of 1400 students. The veterinary curriculum leads to the 'dierenarts' degree (Doctor of Veterinary Medicine, DVM). The veterinary curriculum consists of a three-year bachelor and a three-year master program, specializing in either companion animal, equine, and farm animal/veterinary public health. After completion of the study the veterinarian is generally certified according to Dutch and European law. The 1st year of the master programme started in September 2010.

RESEARCH AND POSTGRADUATE EDUCATION

Research at the faculty of Veterinary Medicine is the responsibility of the Institute for Veterinary Research (IVR). Research which is conducted as part of PhD programmes is linked to one of the research programmes of the IVR. Additionally, all PhD students are participating in Utrecht University's Graduate School of Life Sciences.

QUALITY OF EDUCATION

The faculty of Veterinary Medicine is accredited by the American Veterinary Medical Association (AVMA) and Canadian Veterinary Medical Association (CVMA) since 1973, the European Association of Establishments of Veterinary Education and the Dutch and Flemish Accreditation Organization.

INFORMATION ABOUT THE ADMISSION TO THE FACULTY OF VETERINARY MEDICINE FOR INTERNATIONAL STUDENTS

Special rules apply for the study of Veterinary Medicine. The Dutch Ministry of Education has declared the so-called 'numerus fixes' applicable to the study of Veterinary Medicine. This entails that only 225 students are admitted each year. The number of admission requests largely exceeds the number of allocations. Those restrictions affect both Dutch and international students. The available places are assigned by selection.

ADMISSION

Each year the minister of Education and Science determines the number of students that can be admitted to the study of Veterinary Medicine. At this moment the number is 225. The selection criteria are:

- Average grades at the end-of-5th year pre university education, or the average grades at the end of the 6th year pre university education, or the grades of the final exam after the 6th year pre university education for the mandatory subjects Chemistry, Biology, Physics, Mathematics A or B, Dutch language and English language (30%)

- Result of the knowledge test (30%)

- Result of the "critical reasoning" test (30%)

- Result of the "personality" questionnaire (10%)

Candidates living outside the Netherlands will be offered a validated and secure on-line solution to participate in the selection procedure. For more information, please contact selectie.dgk@uu.nl.

NON-DUTCH DIPLOMAS

Non-Dutch diplomas have to be evaluated and compared with the Dutch equivalent diplomas. This evaluation takes time and can result in the fact that you have to take supplementary exams before being accepted for selection procedure. Information about the evaluation of your diplomas can be obtained at:

Utrecht University, Admissions Office
P.O. Box 80 125, 3508 TC Utrecht, the Netherlands
Phone: +31 30 253 7000
Visiting Address: Heidelberglaan 6, Utrecht – De Uithof

DUTCH LANGUAGE EXAM

Prior to admission to the study of Veterinary Medicine - you have to prove your (sufficient) knowledge of the Dutch language. This is a requirement under the Dutch law because the education is in the Dutch language. The owner of a non-Dutch diploma therefore has to pass the exam "Dutch as Second Language program 2" ('Staatsexamen Nederlands als Tweede Taal, programma 2'), or the Certificate of Dutch as a foreign language 'Certificaat Nederlands als Vreemde Taal: 'Profiel Academische Taalvaardigheid' (PAT) or "Profiel Taalvaardigheid Hoger Onderwijs" (PTHO)' before being admitted. More information about language requirements, courses and examinations can be found through http://www.uu.nl/bachelors/en/limited-enrolment-programmes-dutch under Entry requirements.

TUITION FEES AND SCHOLARSHIPS

The tuition fee depends on your nationality and the programme you register for:

Nationality Programme Tuition 2018-2019

EU/EEA: Bachelor's and Master's programmes: €2,060

Non EU/EEA BSc Veterinary Medicine: €20,767

MSc Veterinary Medicine: €23,882

Information about grants, loans etc. can be found at https://www.uu.nl/bachelors/en/general-information/information-international-students.

RESIDENCE PERMIT

Every international student who wants to receive academic education in the Netherlands needs a residence permit. More information can be obtained at the International Office.

DOCUMENTATION

When requesting admission, the following documents have to be sent to the Admissions Office (see above):

- Your passport copy

- A certified copy of your diploma, OR a certified statement of your school, with the name of the diploma you will obtain and when, and the subjects in which you will be examined

- A certified copy of your transcript

- Official translations of your diploma and transcript (if documents are not in Dutch, English, French, German or Spanish)

- Proof of your proficiency in Dutch

For further information about the admission to the study of Veterinary Medicine please contact:
Study adviser
Faculty of Veterinary Medicine
Department of Educational and Student Affairs
PO Box 80163, 3508 TD Utrecht, the Netherlands
E-mail: osz@vet.uu.nl

Current School Name
University of Illinois at Urbana-Champaign

Why do you want to be a veterinarian?
I am learning that your DVM degree really opens so many doors for you. I not only want the opportunity to make a difference in people's lives by healing their animals, but I also love the fact that I can be a business owner, active in legislation, involved in public health, and so much more. The possibilities with this degree are endless.

What are your short-term and long-term goals?
In the short term, I desperately want to travel abroad. I've never been out of the country and UIUC Vet Med offers so many learning experiences in other countries.

My long-term goals are always changing. As of now, I think I would like to be a practice owner or possibly a board-certified surgeon. Maybe both—who knows!

What did you do as an applicant to prepare for applying to veterinary school?
I tried to set attainable and reasonable goals for myself with my grades, and I gave everything I had in reaching those goals. I indulged in my other hobbies in extracurricular activities (a cappella was my thing), and I tried to be open-minded to different animal experiences. Say yes to things outside of your comfort zone; for me it was semen collection on the university horse farm. It was scary, but I learned and grew from it!

What advice would you give to applicants or those considering applying to veterinary school?
Your very best is the most you can ask of yourself! If you are giving your 100%, stop stressing about the other details. I spent so much time thinking that my best was not good enough, and the truth is that it will be! Take time to live life, too. Well-roundedness and a healthy outlook on life are just as important as your grades when it comes to being an excellent doctor someday!

What helped make the transition to veterinary school easier for you?
I think having a very strong sense of self, and being comfortable in my strengths and weaknesses, has helped me immensely. I chose to take some time off before entering veterinary school, so I'm slightly older than my classmates. That time off gave me time to establish confidence in myself outside of my academics. In vet school, it's so easy to get down on yourself and start to compare yourself to your classmates. Knowing my strengths and capabilities, and being comfortable in working through my weaknesses, has been such an asset in staying sane and focused.

What is your advice on student debt?
What has helped me is keeping my loan money separate from my own earned money. I keep them in two separate accounts and try to only use my loan money for educational costs and the necessities (rent/groceries). This helps me be mindful of how much "fun money" I'm spending, and it has allowed me to have leftover loan money so I can borrow less the following year!

What are you most excited about learning in veterinary school?
Surgery has always fascinated me! I'm really looking forward to junior surgery and the many opportunities to observe the extraordinary surgeons we have here.

VETAGRO SUP*

Email Address: international@vetagro-sup.fr
Website: www.vetagro-sup.fr

VetAgro Sup

SCHOOL DESCRIPTION

VetAgro Sup was born on January 1, 2010 from the merger of the National Veterinary School of Lyon (the oldest veterinary institution established in the world in 1761), the National School of agricultural engineers in Clermont-Ferrand and the National School of Veterinary Services.

Institute of Higher Education and Research in food, animal health, agricultural sciences and the environment, VetAgro Sup operates on both Auvergne and Rhône-Alpes regions and ranks first of its objectives training of veterinarians and engineers, production of knowledge and support for economic, social and public actors in the areas of food, animal health and welfare, agricultural sciences and the environment. VetAgro Sup trains students around multiple veterinary and agricultural occupations (animal health, public health, protection and animal safety, environmental protection, nutrition and food science, etc.).

> VetAgro Sup trains students around multiple veterinary and agricultural occupations.

This great institution was the first French structure created to train both agricultural engineers and veterinary doctors. This model is consistent with international models (university with two colleges), reinforcing the Structure international readability.

With 1,200 students (700 undergraduate vet students) and 120 faculty members gathered in this adventure, VetAgro Sup proposes a set of high-level training in the field of life, legible and competitive national, European and international. The veterinary teaching program is approved by AVMA and EAEVE.

The veterinary campus Lyon (Marcy l'Etoile) and the Agricultural Campus Clermont (Lempdes) are both valued because they offer recognized frameworks for the development of teaching and research. Benefits and services are available to companies and institutional and professional partners: laboratory analysis, medical devices, advice and expertise. Partner authorities (regions Rhône-Alpes and Auvergne, Lyon and Clermont Community, and departments of the Rhone and Puy-de-Dôme) here find a new link for the development of their competitiveness, their scientific potential and their international attractiveness.

FOR INFORMATION ON APPLYING TO VETAGRO SUP:

VetAgro Sup
College of Veterinary Medicine
1 Avenue Bourgelat
69280 Marcy L'Etoile, FRANCE
Phone: 04 78 87 25 25
Email: international@vetagro-sup.fr
Website: http://www.vetagro-sup.fr

AAVMC AFFILIATE MEMBER
VETERINARY MEDICAL SCHOOLS
Non-COE Accredited

UNIVERSITY OF ADELAIDE

Email: avs_enquiries@adelaide.edu.au
Website: www.adelaide.edu.au

THE UNIVERSITY
of ADELAIDE

SCHOOL DESCRIPTION

The School of Animal and Veterinary Sciences at the University of Adelaide is located in South Australia. The University of Adelaide is a world-class tertiary education and research institution committed to delivering high-quality and distinct learning, teaching and research experiences. The University was established in 1874 and is consistently ranked in the top 1% of universities worldwide. It is a member of the Group of Eight, a coalition of Australia's foremost research intensive universities. The University constitutes a vibrant and diverse community with over 25,000 students and over 3,500 members of staff across our three main campuses (North Terrace, Roseworthy and Waite).

> The University of Adelaide is is consistently ranked in the top 1% of universities worldwide.

The School of Animal and Veterinary Sciences is based at the Roseworthy Campus, which is located approximately 30 miles (50 kilometres) north of Adelaide. Australia's first agricultural college was established at Roseworthy, in 1883. Since its establishment, the Australian agricultural industry has recognised Roseworthy Agricultural College as the premier teaching facility for the sector and close partnerships with industry and government research groups have always been a feature of Roseworthy's development. In 1991, the Roseworthy Agricultural College joined forces with the University of Adelaide. The Bachelor of Science (BSc) (Animal Science) has been taught at the campus since 2004 and the veterinary program commenced in 2008.

Roseworthy Campus is located on a 1600 ha property and includes a working farm on which students gain practical experience and training. In addition, our leading-edge Veterinary Health Centre (which includes the Companion Animal Health Centre, Equine Health and Performance Centre, Production Animal Health Centre and Veterinary Diagnostic Laboratories), provides exceptional services to the public and offers students in the Doctor of Veterinary Medicine (DVM) program real-world experience.

The campus is currently home to over 100 staff and approximately 650 students, including undergraduates, and post-graduates in both coursework and higher degree by research (Masters and PhD). The campus is a vibrant and exciting centre for undergraduate teaching, post-graduate training and clinical service and is fast becoming the major animal and veterinary research centre for the State.

PROGRAM OVERVIEW

At the University of Adelaide, the veterinary science program is comprised of two degrees: the BSc (Veterinary Bioscience) and the DVM. Students satisfactorily completing the undergraduate degree will gain direct entry into the postgraduate program and completion of both degrees (6 years in total) is required to register as a veterinarian.

The veterinary science program at the University of Adelaide has been granted accreditation by the Australasian Veterinary Boards Council (AVBC), the Veterinary Surgeons' Board of Hong Kong, and the Royal College of Veterinary Surgeons (UK). Graduates from this program are eligible for registration as veterinarians in all states and territories of Australia, New Zealand, Hong Kong, Singapore, South Africa and the United

Kingdom. The program also has affiliation membership with the Association of American Veterinary Medical Colleges.

APPLICATION INFORMATION

For specific application information please email avs_enquiries@adelaide.edu.au.

Residency implications: 60 domestic (Commonwealth supported places) and 20 international places.

Required academic grades:

Bachelor of Science (Veterinary Bioscience) – International Applicants

Academic entry requirements for standard qualifications are as follows:

- Australian Tertiary Admissions Rank (ATAR) – minimum 90
- International Baccalaureate (IB) – minimum 31
- Grade Point Average (GPA) – minimum of 5.0 (on a 7.0 scale)
- SAT (US) – minimum 1410

Other qualifications, including international qualifications, will be considered on their individual merits; further information is available through the degree finder on the University of Adelaide website (https://www.adelaide.edu.au/degree-finder/2018/bscpv_bscaspv.html).

Course completion deadline: Prerequisite courses must be completed by 31st December.

Doctor of Veterinary Medicine – International Applicants
- Minimum GPA: 5.0 on a 7.0 scale

Credit policy: Students may be credited with advanced standing (status/exemption) for courses already completed at another institution and therefore may be eligible for entry into 2nd year of the BSc (Veterinary Bioscience) or 1st year of the DVM. Courses must appear on official college transcripts and be equivalent to the corresponding courses at the University of Adelaide.

Course completion deadline: Prerequisite courses must be completed by 31 December.

ADDITIONAL REQUIREMENTS AND CONSIDERATIONS

Supplemental application required:

Bachelor of Science (Veterinary Bioscience) – International Applicants

Prescribed questionnaire: To gain entry into the BSc (Veterinary Bioscience) program, applicants should be able to demonstrate an informed interest in veterinary science, animals and their welfare, and articulate a clear understanding of, and commitment to, the breadth and intensity of training which is required in a veterinary program.

Applicants must submit the Prescribed questionnaire and supporting statements (including references) by the closing date. The questionnaire includes the following components:
- Details of animal husbandry and veterinary experiences
- Personal statement demonstrating their interest in a career in the veterinary profession, references
- Extracurricular and community service activities.

Doctor of Veterinary Medicine – International Applicants

Applicants must submit to the University the Self-Assessment Checklist on skills learned in extramural studies accompanied by a 1-2 page description of how these skills were acquired.

Inherent Requirements:

There are inherent requirements associated with the BSc (Veterinary Bioscience) and DVM programs that prospective students need to be aware of before applying. Further details can be found at https://www.adelaide.edu.au/degree-finder/2018/dvetm_drvetmedi.html

SUMMARY OF ADMISSIONS PROCEDURES

Prerequisite information

Bachelor of Science (Veterinary Bioscience) – International Applicants

Mathematics and Chemistry

English Language Requirements (if applicable)

Doctor of Veterinary Medicine – International Applicants

BSc (Veterinary Bioscience) from the University of Adelaide or equivalent.

English Language Requirements (if applicable)

ADMISSION INFORMATION

Bachelor of Science (Veterinary Bioscience) – International Applicants

Application deadlines: Applications can be received on an ongoing basis throughout the year. The final deadline is 30th September.

Interview dates: Questionnaires will be assessed as soon as possible after submission and eligible applicants will be invited to participate in an online interview. Dates and times for the interview will be negotiated between the School and the applicant.

Date acceptances mailed: Allow 2 weeks once final academic results have been received and interviews have been conducted.

School begins: March

Deposit: $9,000

Deferments: Up to one year

Transfer students: Yes

Evaluation Criteria: Selection for the interview process will be based on the assessment of the questionnaire. Applicants who are successful in gaining an interview will be ranked for an offer, based on a combination of scores from the following two components:

Academic Results: 50%
Interview Results: 50%

Doctor of Veterinary Medicine – International Applicants

Application Deadlines: Application can be receive on an ongoing basis throughout the year. The final deadline is 30th September.

Date acceptances mailed: Allow 2 weeks once final academic results have been received and Self-Assessment Checklist has been reviewed.

School begins: March

Deposit: $9,000

Deferments: Up to one year

Transfer students: Yes

Evaluation Criteria: Applicants academic transcript, grades and Self-Assessment Checklist will be assessed to determine if they are eligible and will be ranked based on their academic grades.

2017 ADMISSIONS SUMMARY

Number of applicants:

	BSc (Veterinary Bioscience)	DVM
Domestic	427	51 from BSc + 14 external
International	26	6
Total	453	71

Number of new entrants:

	BSc (Veterinary Bioscience)	DVM
Domestic	60	53
International	3	6
Total	63	59

EXPENSES FOR THE 2016 ACADEMIC YEAR

Tuition & Fees:

Bachelor of Science (Veterinary Bioscience)

Domestic Students (Commonwealth supported place): $10,125 per year

International Students: $59,000 per year

Doctor of Veterinary Medicine

Domestic Students (Commonwealth supported place): $10,750 per year

International Students: $59,000 per year

Scholarships: Information regarding International student scholarships can be found at https://international.adelaide.edu.au/admissions/scholarships-sponsorships

ENTRANCE REQUIREMENTS

Admitted students fall into two categories: Domestic (Commonwealth supported place) and International. Applicants must verify their residency status on application.

CENTRAL LUZON STATE UNIVERSITY*

Email Address: clsu@clsu.edu.ph
Website: clsucvsm.edu.ph

SCHOOL DESCRIPTION

Central Luzon State University (CLSU) is located on a 658-hectare sprawling main campus in the Science City of Muñoz, which is located 150 kilometers north of Manila. It also has a more than 1000-hectare site for ranch type buffalo production and forestry development up the hills of Carranglan town, in northern Nueva Ecija, 40 kilometers away from the main campus. The University is the lead agency of the Muñoz Science Community and the seat of the Regional Research and Development Center in Central Luzon. To date, CLSU is one of the premier institutions of agriculture in Southeast Asia known for its breakthrough researches in aquaculture (pioneer in the sex reversal of Tilapia), ruminants, crops, orchard, and water management researches.

> For many years, DVM graduates from CVSM have consistently topped the Veterinary Licensure Examinations in the country.

The College of Veterinary Science and Medicine (CVSM) was established in 1978 through Republic Act No. 4067 enacted into law by Congress in 1964. Subsequently, CVSM offered the first ladderized veterinary curriculum in the Philippines: Bachelor of Science in Animal Husbandry (first 4 years) and Doctor of Veterinary Medicine (6 years). This was designed to produce veterinarians adept not only in disease control and prevention but in animal production as well. For many years, DVM graduates from CVSM have consistently topped the Veterinary Licensure Examinations in the country. This excellent performance has made the Philippine Commission on Higher Education (CHED) and the Professional Regulation Commission (PRC) to recognize the CVSM as one of the Top Performing Veterinary Colleges in the country. In 2009, CHED awarded the college the title, Center of Excellence in Veterinary Medicine.

APPLICATION INFORMATION

The following are the admission requirements for both undergraduate and graduate programs:

UNDERGRADUATE PROGRAM

1. Must have a GPA of 2.25 or better. Second courser must have at least 2.50 or better.
2. Must have taken a minimum of 40 units of general education courses.
3. Must not have a grade of "5".
4. Grades of "4" or "INC" must be removed or completed upon filing of application.
5. Must qualify in the online exam and panel interview conducted by the college admission committee.
6. Submission of duly accomplished application form with:
   A. four (4) 2x2 pictures (studio taken only)
   B. certification of grades (1st and 2nd semester)

For Transferees
1. Applicants must meet all the prescribed admission requirements of the University/College and the course applied for:
   a. Must qualify in the University/College Admission Test
   b. Must have complete and valid credentials
      (a) Copy of birth certificate
      (b) Two 2"x2" colored ID pictures

(c) Certificate of completion of a secondary curriculum

(d) Original transcript of records

(e) Personal history statement

(f) Affidavit of support

(g) Alien certificate of registration (ACR)

(h) Student visa

(i) Certificate of Proficiency in English issued by the CLSU Department of English and Humanities for a fee, for students who come from countries where English is not the medium of instruction

(j) Security clearance from his/her embassy

c. Must pay a non-refundable application fee

d. Must qualify in the physical or health examination conducted by the University physician

e. Must present an approved application for admission

f. Others as prescribed by the concerned College

2. Applicants must meet all the prescribed requirements by the Department of Foreign Affairs and the BID.

3. A foreign student may be admitted based on availability of slot in the course applied for.

4. He or she must pledge to abide by and comply with the rules and regulations of the University/College.

GRADUATE PROGRAM

A DVM degree or its equivalent from a recognized institution is a requirement along with the submission of the following:

1. Duly accomplished application form

2. Original or authenticated transcript of records showing a grade point average (GPA) of at least 2.0 or its equivalent.

3. Applicants with GPA below 2.0 may be admitted on a probationary status if recommended by the department chair and approved by the dean after thorough review of the applicant's qualification to do graduate work.

4. Two letters of recommendation from former professors in the undergraduate course.

Is a Bachelor's Degree Required? no

Is this an International School? yes

ESTIMATED TUITION

Estimated Tuition Resident: Php 7,000.00 per semester

Estimated Tuition Non-Resident (International): Php 12,000.00 per semester

AVAILABLE SEATS

Resident: N/A

Non-Resident (International): n/a

VMCAS Participation: non-VMCAS

Accepts International Students? yes

Application Deadline: Last week of April every year.

UNIVERSITY OF COPENHAGEN*

Email: hhd@sund.ku.dk
Website: www.sund.ku.dk

UNIVERSITY OF
COPENHAGEN

SCHOOL DESCRIPTION

The Veterinary School in Copenhagen was founded in 1773 as one of the first schools in the world. In 1856 the veterinary school was moved to its present location and at that time acquired the status of an institution of higher learning incorporating agriculture and animal science. In 2007 the Royal Veterinary and Agricultural University merged with the University of Copenhagen and was transformed into the Faculty of Life Sciences incorporating the veterinary school. The University of Copenhagen was inaugurated on 1 June 1479, after King Christian I was granted approval for its establishment by Pope Sixtus IV. Based on a German model, the university consisted of four faculties: Theology, Law, Medicine and Philosophy. Today with more than 38,000 students and more than 9,000 employees, the University of Copenhagen is the largest institution of research and education in Denmark. The purpose of the University – to quote the University Statute – is to 'conduct research and provide further education to the highest academic level'.

> The University of Copenhagen is the largest institution of research and education in Denmark.

Approximately one hundred different institutes, departments, laboratories, centers, museums, etc., form the nucleus of the University, where professors, lecturers and other academic staff, as well as most of the technical and administrative personnel, carry out their daily work, and where teaching takes place. With the opening of the totally rebuilt and modernized Small Animal University Hospital at the Frederiksberg Campus in early 2011 the Copenhagen Veterinary School including the newly built Large Animal University Hospital at the Taastrup Campus functions as one of the most modern veterinary schools with state of the art equipment.

In 2012 the Copenhagen School of Veterinary Medicine together with the School of Pharmaceutical Sciences merged with the Faculty of Health to form a new, scientifically and financially strong Faculty of Health and Medicine within the University of Copenhagen.

ORGANIZATION AND STAFF

The veterinary school encompasses 2 departments with specialized facilities, a Faculty Office and a number of general services (e.g., learning environment with audiovisual units, library, experimental farms, student facilities including several computer rooms, etc). The veterinary school has an academic staff of 276 academic staff, including 29 full professors and an administrative and support staff of 356 support staff. Most staff members communicate well in English and all academic staff members have experience in teaching veterinary medicine in English. In early 2012 all academic staff members have completed officially approved proficiency tests in English.

UNDERGRADUATE VETERINARY EDUCATION

Admission of students to the 5½-year undergraduate veterinary training program is limited to 180 each year, resulting in a total of 1100 students. They pass full examinations at the completion of each course.

RESEARCH AND POSTGRADUATE EDUCATION

Research at the School of Veterinary Medicine is the responsibility of the Vice Dean for Research and the department heads. Research which is conducted as part of the PhD programs is included in this portfolio.

QUALITY OF EDUCATION

The School of Veterinary Medicine, Faculty of Health and Medicine within the University of Copenhagen has been regularly evaluated and accredited by the European Association of Establishments of Veterinary Education since 1988 (latest accreditation in 2010).

INFORMATION ABOUT THE ADMISSION TO THE FACULTY OF VETERINARY MEDICINE FOR FOREIGN STUDENTS

In general foreign students have access to the Danish universities.

Special rules apply for the study of Veterinary Medicine. The Danish Ministry of Science has declared a numerous clauses to the DVM program. This entails that only a limited amount of students is admitted each year. The number of admission requests largely exceeds the number of allocations. Restrictions affect both Danish and foreign students. The available places are assigned by selection through interviews (50%) or based upon grades obtained in high school (50%). Letters of recommendation are neither required nor accepted.

APPLICATION TO THE DANISH DVM PROGRAM

Each year the minister of education and science lays down the number of students to be admitted to the DVM program. Currently 180 students are accepted in each class. There are two routes of application. The first is solely based upon high school grades (Quota I) and the second is based upon a mixture of high school grades, working experience and an interview (Quota II). No standardized tests are required before application. Application deadline for Quota I is 5 July 2015, and for Quota II the application deadline is 15 March 2017.

International students are referred to http://vetschool.ku.dk/english for further information about application for the Danish DVM program.

TUITION FEES AND SCHOLARSHIPS

Generally students from within the European Union do not pay tuition fee. For foreign students please refer to web site of the Ministry of Science, Technology and Innovation http://en.vtu.dk or to http://vetschool.ku.dk/english. Generally financial aid is not offered to foreign students.

RESIDENCE PERMIT

Foreign students who want to receive an academic education in Denmark need a residence permit. More information can be obtained at the Danish embassy in the country of origin.

Additionally applicants must demonstrate access to sufficient financial means. The amount varies and more detailed information should be sought at a Danish embassy.

PRE-VETERINARY PROFILE: EMMA WALSH

Current School Name
Hamilton College

What type of veterinary medicine are you interested in pursuing, and why?
I am interested in becoming a general practitioner at a small animal clinic or dealing with exotic animals. These interests are inspired by my dealings with animals throughout life.

What is/was your major during undergraduate school?
My intended major is biology with a minor in philosophy.

What are your short-term and long-term goals?
Short-term, I would like to gain as much veterinary experience as I can, especially with large animals outside clinics. Long-term, I would love to someday work in a shelter, helping make dogs, cats, and other species more adoptable.

What are you doing as an applicant/pre-vet to prepare for veterinary school?
To prepare for veterinary school I am gaining as much experience as I can with animals, especially observing surgeries in clinics.

What extracurricular activities are you involved in currently?
Currently I am involved in the Hunt and Dressage Club, Vegan Club, the Pre-Health Club, and 4-H. I also recently started shadowing at a local clinic.

How old were you when you first became interested in being a veterinarian?
I don't remember my exact age, but I was always fascinated with animals, and when I realized that helping them was a viable career option, I decided that was what I wanted to do.

Please describe your various experiences in preparation for applying to veterinary school.
Though I am still very early in the process, I have found that taking as many science courses as possible is a wise course of action. Seeking advice from any veterinarians is also very helpful.

What characteristics are you looking for in a veterinary school?
In a veterinary school I am looking for a willingness to work closely with students, opportunities for research that I find interesting, a focus on the animals, and a chance to study abroad.

What advice do you have for other pre-veterinary students?
I would advise getting as much experience as possible as soon as possible and devoting a lot of time to schoolwork. I would also suggest balancing pre-vet requirements with exploratory classes in completely unrelated subjects and doing any extracurricular activities that you find interesting, not just those that relate to veterinary medicine.

SEOUL NATIONAL UNIVERSITY*

Email Address: snuadmit@snu.ac.kr
Website: en.snu.ac.kr/apply/info

서 울 대 학 교
SEOUL NATIONAL UNIVERSITY

SCHOOL DESCRIPTION

Seoul National University honors the ideals of liberal education and aims to teach students a lifelong love of learning that will form the basis for continuous personal growth.

At the same time it is committed to preparing students to work and live in an increasingly competitive global environment. As South Korea's first national university, Seoul National University has a tradition of standing up for democracy and peace on the Korean peninsula.

Graduates have long served as public servants in key positions of the Korean government. In teaching, research, and public service, Seoul National University continues to set the standard of excellence.

The mission of Seoul National University in the twenty-first century is to create a vibrant intellectual community where students and scholars join together in building the future. As Korea's leading research university, Seoul National University is committed to diversifying its student body and faculty, fostering global exchange, and promoting path-breaking research in all fields of knowledge.

> In teaching, research, and public service, Seoul National University continues to set the standard of excellence.

2016 FALL ADMISSIONS TIMELINE

The dates and deadlines below are for the application to the program that starts in Fall 2016

ONLINE APPLICATION

Period : January 11 (Mon)~February 18 (Thu), 2016
  *Note that the entrance to the program is in Sep, 2016.

SUBMISSION OF DOCUMENTS

Period: January 11 (Mon)~February 29 (Fri), 2016
  *After completing the online application, the required documents should arrive at the SNU Office of Admissions by due date.

PERFORMANCE TEST

International admission type II (Undergraduate) applicant who received the entire education abroad applying for the following programs: Fine Arts, Music, or Physical Education, may be subject to a performance test.
  *In such a case, the corresponding College/Department will individually notify the applicants for futher details.

ANNOUNCEMENT OF ADMISSIONS DECISION

April 27 (Wed), 2016
  *Results will be posted on the SNU website NOTICE

REGISTRATION

August 2016 (TBA)
  *Either at the branches of NongHyup Bank, Shinhan Bank, Woori Bank nationwide or via virtual account transfer

KOREAN PROFICIENCY TEST AMONG THE ADMITTED STUDENTS

August 2016 (TBA)
  SNU website will indicate those who are required to take the Korean proficiency Test on the admission result announcement screen.

• For further information about application process and admissions, please make an inquiry to Office of admissions' email address. (snuadmit@snu.ac.kr) or (http://en.snu.ac.kr/apply/info)

ST. MATTHEW'S UNIVERSITY

Email Address: admissions@stmatthews.edu
Website: www.stmatthews.edu

SCHOOL DESCRIPTION

St. Matthew's University School of Veterinary Medicine is located on beautiful Grand Cayman in the Caribbean. Grand Cayman is the fifth largest financial district in the world and has a highly developed infrastructure which is very comparable to the United States. It is also one of the safest islands in the Caribbean, boasting one of the lowest crime and poverty rates. Grand Cayman has hundreds of restaurants, scores of banks, world-class hotels, and many opportunities for boating, diving, horseback riding, and other recreation. The island is less than an hours flight from Miami, and also has direct flights from Atlanta, Chicago, Charlotte, Houston, Tampa, Toronto, Washington D.C., and other locations.

> Throughout your ten semesters at St. Matthew's University, we will support all aspects of your education and life.

At SMU, we are as committed to your dreams as you are. Throughout your ten semesters with us, we will do everything we can to ensure your success by supporting all aspects of your education and life, including:

Focus on Teaching: Dedicated, talented faculty whose time commitments are focused on teaching and mentoring.

Student Mentors: Student mentors understand about adjusting to life in veterinary school, and are eager to see you succeed.

Very Low Student to Faculty Ratio: With a student to faculty ratio of less than four to one, you will have an unprecedented level of faculty support and attention.

We limit each incoming cohort of students to a maximum of 20.

Best Value: Most affordable tuition of any Caribbean veterinary school.

Graduate in 3+ Years: Complete your pre-clinical education on Grand Cayman in just 28 months, and then return to the U.S. or Canada for clinical training, with the ability to complete vet school in just over three years.

SMU's modern, state-of-the-art main campus is located across the street from beautiful Seven Mile Beach, and boasts wireless technology throughout the bright, air-conditioned classrooms, labs, library, and student lounges. SMU also has a Clinical Teaching Facility which hosts surgery, medicine and clinical skills training as well as anatomy and pathology laboratories. Students have the opportunity to travel to local farms with veterinary staff from the Cayman Department of Agriculture. Our students spend seven (7) semesters on Grand Cayman and their final months in clinical programs at one of our many AVMA-accredited Clinical Program Affiliate Schools in the United States and Canada.

There arc significant opportunities for students to gain experience with exotic species through our collaborations with the Cayman Turtle Farm, Central Caribbean Marine Institute, Dolphin Discovery, the Blue Iguana Project, and the Marine Research Program.

APPLICATION INFORMATION

We welcome applications from any qualified candidate who dreams of become a veterinarian. For specific application information (availability, deadlines, fees, transferring to SMU and VMCAS participation), please refer to the contact information above.

SUMMARY OF ADMISSIONS PROCEDURES

Timetable

Application deadlines: None. Rolling admissions. Three incoming cohorts per year.

Interviews: Held in person or via videoconference.

School begins: August, January, May (three start dates per year).

Deposit (to hold a place in class): $500.00

Deferments: Considered on an individual basis.

Transfer applications for admission with advanced standings are welcome. Transfer credits (advance standing) may be awarded at the discretion of the University.

Seats generally available: Maximum of 20 (total) seats available per incoming cohort to ensure exceptional level of faculty support for students.

ENTRANCE REQUIREMENTS

All prerequisite courses must be completed prior to matriculation.

Is a Bachelor's Degree Required? no

Is this an International School? yes

ESTIMATED TUITION

Estimated Tuition Resident: Pre-Clinical Sciences (Grand Cayman): $15,125

Estimated Tuition Contract: Clinical Sciences (Clinical Affiliates): $23,000

Estimated Tuition Non-Resident: Additional Fees: $0

AVAILABLE SEATS

Resident: 0

Contract: 0

Non-Resident: 20, 3 times per year

TEST REQUIREMENTS

Graduate Record Examination (GRE), general test, is not required but is recommended.

VMCAS Participation: non-VMCAS

Accepts International Students? yes

ADDITIONAL INFORMATION

The admissions team at SMU wants to get to know you! To us, you are much more than a GPA or GRE score. We want to know about you as a person because ultimately, that is what will determine the kind of veterinarian you will be. We want to support you in your dream of becoming a veterinarian, and we welcome your application!

Application Deadline: rolling

UNIVERSITY OF TOKYO*

Graduate School of Agricultural and Life Sciences
The University of Tokyo
1-1-1, Yayoi, Bunkyo-ku, Tokyo, 113-8657

SCHOOL DESCRIPTION

Veterinary medicine covers wide areas of life sciences, not only medicine for animals but also biology of mammals and higher vertebrates. In the Department of Veterinary Medicine, most advanced research is being carried out at molecular, cellular and in vivo levels, in order to fully understand vital processes of normal and diseased animals. Veterinary medicine has two aspects of science: basic science to understand the mechanisms underlying biological phenomena, and applied science to satisfy the social demands for maintenance and improvement of human welfare and productivity of domestic animals. This department collaborates with the veterinary medical center located on the Yayoi campus. This center is facilitated with the latest and most advanced medical instruments, and plays an important role as an advanced veterinary hospital in this area.

> The Department of Veterinary Medicine collaborates with the veterinary medical center located on the Yayoi campus.

FOR MORE INFORMATION

For more information about the University of Tokyo's Veterinary Medicine Program, please go to the following website: http://www.u-tokyo.ac.jp/en/admissions-and-programs/graduate-and-research/graduate-schools/agricultural.html

UNITED ARAB EMIRATES UNIVERSITY*

Email Address: servicedesk@uaeu.ac.ae
Website: www.uaeu.ac.ae/en/catalog/undergraduate
/programs/program_21931.shtml

 جامعة الإمارات العربية المتحدة
United Arab Emirates University

SCHOOL DESCRIPTION

The Bachelor of Veterinary Medicine Program is the only one of its kind in the United Arab Emirates. The program is five years long, after which graduates will be qualified veterinarians. Students will receive veterinary basic sciences education and intensive clinical training sorted by animal species and specialized disciplines.

> The Bachelor of Veterinary Medicine Program is the only one of its kind in the United Arab Emirates.

PROGRAM OBJECTIVES

The Bachelor of Veterinary Medicine Program at UAE University aims to: enable the veterinary students to acquire knowledge, practical skills, and experience needed for a qualified veterinarian; enforce evidence-based veterinary medicine and problem-oriented, problem solving methods; graduate veterinarians capable of providing superior animal health care, including disease investigation and prevention, at the individual and herd or flock level; meet the growing national needs for qualified veterinarians in the public and private sectors; and demonstrate the achievement of the PLOs by the graduation time and enable graduates to pursue higher academic degrees in veterinary medical sciences or other related sciences.

FOR MORE INFORMATION

For more information about the Bachelor's of Veterinary Medicine Program at UAE University, please go to the following website: https://www.uaeu.ac.ae/en/catalog/undergraduate/programs/program_21931.shtml

For information about admissions into the University, please go to: https://www.uaeu.ac.ae/en/admission

UNIVERSITY OF VETERINARY AND ANIMAL SCIENCES, LAHORE-PAKISTAN*

Email Address: webmaster@uvas.edu.pk
Website: www.uvas.edu.pk/index.php

LAHORE

SCHOOL DESCRIPTION

With a marvelous history of 133 years of excellence, the University of Veterinary and Animal Sciences (UVAS), Lahore, is now positioned among the top ten Universities of Pakistan. Originally established as a school in 1882, it was later transformed into a college within the next two decades (i.e., end of the nineteenth century). Realizing the importance of livestock and poultry sectors in the economy of the country and the growing need of human resource and research work in veterinary and animal sciences and allied fields in the country, this historic institution was upgraded as a university in 2002. Presently, UVAS comprises of 23 departments in five faculties, three institutes, one constituent college, and a school, along with seven affiliated institutes at Attock, Rawalpindi, Shiekhupura, Okara, Lahore, Narowal, and Sahiwal.

> With a marvelous history of 133 years of excellence, UVAS is positioned among the top ten universities of Pakistan.

The UVAS reflects a unique blend of glorious history and ongoing professional advancement of the modern era. The main building of the institution, which was built 100 years ago, is still considered as the symbol of historical glory while the University has now expanded to five campuses, including its City Campus Lahore, Ravi Campus Pattoki, Avian Research & Training Center at Ferozepur Road, College of Veterinary and Animal Sciences Jhang, and the Para Veterinary School in Karor Lal Easin, District Layyah.

FOR MORE INFORMATION

For more information about the University of Veterinary and Animal Science-Pakistan's DMV program, please go to the following website: http://www.uvas.edu.pk/Admissions/undergraduate/DVM/

VETERINARIAN PROFILE: CONRAD SPANGLER

YEAR OF GRADUATION
2009

PLACE OF EMPLOYMENT
Riverview, LLP

What is your favorite aspect of being a veterinarian?
My favorite aspect of a being a veterinarian is the people I get to work with on a daily basis. The clients and caretakers of the dairy cows and calves I work with are hard-working, honest people who want the best for their families, communities, the environment, and the animals they care for. I have learned so much from them about life and animal care.

What type of veterinary medicine do you practice?
I practice dairy production medicine for a private dairy production company, Riverview, LLP.

Where did you attend veterinary school?
University of Minnesota.

How long have you been practicing as a veterinarian?
Eight years.

What advice do you have for those considering a career in veterinary medicine?
Understand the financial realities of a career in veterinary medicine and do some deep introspection to decide if you are passionate enough about this career path to overcome the financial difficulties you will face upon leaving veterinary school. Veterinary schools are admitting more students and charging them more to make up for a lack of funding, which has the potential to oversupply veterinarians and push wages down. The net present value for a veterinary education is negative for many practice types, which means it is potentially a bad investment for many students. Be sure to balance the emotional excitement of veterinary school with the financial realities and determine if you have the fortitude to truly succeed in this business.

What challenges have you faced while practicing veterinary medicine?
The two main challenges I have faced while practicing veterinary medicine are repaying student loan debt and learning how to work with and motivate clients to change. The amount of student loan debt has the potential to force one to put off other major investments in order to repay the loans, which can make savings for retirement, home ownership, and children challenging. Additionally, it can be frustrating when clients don't follow your recommendations. It is important to learn you can't be everything to everybody, and you need to adjust your strategy to motivate different personality types in order to achieve compliance with your recommendations.

POLICIES ON ADVANCED STANDING

Transfers are permitted to most colleges of veterinary medicine in the United States under specified conditions. Typical requirements include a vacancy in the class, completion of all prerequisite requirements, and compatible curricula. Following is a listing of schools and some of the conditions under which they will consider a transfer from another veterinary college with advanced standing. More detailed information may be obtained by writing to the individual schools in which you have an interest.

UNITED STATES

UNIVERSITY OF CALIFORNIA, DAVIS

Applications may be considered if available positions exist within the third-year class.

1. The applicant must have a strong academic record in their undergraduate program. At minimum, the candidate's application score used for the regular admissions process must meet or exceed the average application score for the class in which the candidate is seeking admission. This is the quantitative measure used to rank applicants—it is based on a combination of quantitative data including GPA (overall VMCAS science courses, and most recent 45 graded semester units), GRE quantitative score, and quantitative input from external letters. The average overall science GPA is 3.7; most recent 45 semester units is 3.8; 74% is the quantitative GRE.

2. The applicant must be currently enrolled in an AVMA-accredited DVM program and must be in excellent academic and ethical standing in that program. The specific minimum benchmark will be that the applicant is in the top quartile of students in the Veterinary School in which the applicant is currently enrolled as determined by GPA or class rank.

3. The applicant must have completed veterinary course work equivalent to that expected of the students in the DVM program of the School of Veterinary Medicine, UC Davis, who will be in the same academic class.

4. The applicant has a valid reason for requesting admission in advanced standing.

UNIVERSITY OF FLORIDA

1. An opening must exist in the second- or third-year class.

2. Students are only rarely considered for advanced standing based on exceptional personal circumstances.

3. Student must be enrolled in an AVMA accredited college.

4. Student must meet all prerequisites for admission as a first-year student (including GRE® scores).

5. The curricula of the two schools must be sufficiently alike to allow a student to enter without deficiencies in academic background.

6. Applicants must have a letter approving transfer from their dean or associate dean.

UNIVERSITY OF GEORGIA

1. Priority is given to Georgia residents, followed by contract state residents, then all other applicants.

2. Applicants will be considered for entry into the DVM degree program up to the third year of the curriculum, when and if space is available, as defined by the Admissions Committee.

3. Applications must include official transcripts of all completed veterinary and pre-veterinary coursework and a letter of support written by a senior administrator of the school in which the applicant is currently enrolled stating the applicant is currently in good academic standing.

4. No individual is eligible for transfer who has been dismissed or is on probation at any other school or college for deficiency in scholarship or because of misconduct.

UNIVERSITY OF ILLINOIS

1. Transfer students will only be considered for the beginning of the second year of veterinary medicine and only if transfer seats become available in that class.

2. All prerequisite science courses must be completed prior to the request for transfer.

3. Minimum grade requirements include:
   cumulative and science GPAs of 2.75 on a 4.00 scale (doesn't include veterinary work); results of the Graduate Record Examination General Test completed within the last two years.

4. Student must complete the same preveterinary coursework as required for students accepted to the first year of the program.

5. Student must be in good academic standing.

6. To be considered for transfer, a student must present credentials for preprofessional work that ful-

fill the University of Illinois College of Veterinary Medicine requirements for first-year entry.

7. Complete information and an application can be found at http://vetmed.illinois.edu/education/doctor -veterinary-medicine-degree/transfer-information

COLORADO STATE UNIVERSITY

Transfer is dependent on position openings in the year into which the student transfers (most transfers usually involve the loss of a year because of differences in school curricula). Candidate must:

1. have successfully completed at least the first year (equivalent of two semesters) of veterinary curriculum at an AVMA accredited college of veterinary medicine and be currently enrolled at the time of request.

AND

2. have obtained the equivalent of a 3.0 cumulative GPA in your veterinary program AND must not have received a D, F, or unsatisfactory grade of any kind at any time since enrolling in veterinary school.

AND

3. have a preveterinary academic record comparable to currently enrolled DVM students.

AND

4. provide evidence of noncognitive attributes comparable to currently enrolled DVM students.

5. A student who is accepted for transfer may be required to successfully complete Capstone Examinations associated with the class year into which they are transferring.

If a veterinary student with an interest in transferring to CSU's DVM program meets ALL of the above minimum requirements, he/she may apply to the DVM program. To apply for transfer to CSU's Veterinary Program, please see http://csu-cvmbs.colostate.edu/dvm -program/Pages/dvm-transfer-student-opportunities .aspx

CORNELL UNIVERSITY

1. Students are considered for advanced standing on an individual basis.
2. Transfer students will be considered if an opening exists in the second-year class. Students seeking advanced standing may enter the DVM program at two points: at the beginning of the second year of study, or mid-way through the second year, at the beginning of the fourth (Spring) semester of study.
3. Students seeking advanced standing must be enrolled in an AVMA-accredited veterinary college.

4. The curricula of the two schools must be sufficiently similar to allow students to enter without deficiencies in their academic background.
5. Students must meet all pre-veterinary requirements for first-year entry at the College of Veterinary Medicine at Cornell University (including GRE scores, prerequisite coursework, animal and veterinary experience), and may not have any failing grades on their veterinary transcript.
6. Scores from the Graduate Record Examination (GRE) or Medical College Admissions Test (MCAT) may not be older than five years.
7. Applicants seeking advanced standing must include a letter from their Associate Dean certifying that the student is in good academic standing, has not been on academic probation, and has not been subject to any disciplinary action or dismissal for any reason.
8. Applicants are required to have completed at least two full semesters at the institution from which the transfer is requested. Only veterinary coursework completed at an AVMA-accredited institution will be considered.
9. After analyzing the academic background of the applicant, the Admissions Committee will place each accepted transfer student in the semester of study in the DVM curriculum deemed most appropriate. (Veterinary course syllabi will be required at time of application).

IOWA STATE UNIVERSITY

Acceptance of students for advanced standing is on the recommendation of the Academic Standards Committee. Space must be available in the class to which the student is applying. See website, http://vetmed.iastate .edu/student/future-dvm-students/apply-to-the-college /transfer-admissions/application-process.

KANSAS STATE UNIVERSITY

Acceptance of students for transfer is on recommendation of the Admissions Committee on a space-available basis. Further information is available at http://www .vet.k-state.edu/admissions/apply/transfer-app.html

LINCOLN MEMORIAL UNIVERSITY

Transfer students are considered. Each applicant is evaluated on an individual basis. Potential transfer students can find additional information regarding LMU-CVM at the following link: https://www.lmunet.edu /academics/schools/college-of-veterinary-medicine /admissions/transfer-policy

LOUISIANA STATE UNIVERSITY

1. Transfer applications are considered on a case-by-case and space available basis.
2. The curricula must be compatible and how many semesters a student must have at their current school will be based on this compatibility.
3. The student must be in good academic standing with at least a 3.2 GPA in veterinary coursework at his/her present school.
4. Admission is limited to the second year of the program and only into the fall semester.
5. Applicants requesting a transfer must contact the Office of Veterinary Education and Student Affairs. They must be currently enrolled and in good standing and their present school must be aware of their intent to transfer. A letter of good standing will be needed as part of the transfer documentation.
6. To initiate the transfer process, please carefully read the DVM Transfer Guidelines information at http://www.lsu.edu/vetmed/dvm_admissions/how_to_apply/transfers.php.

MICHIGAN STATE UNIVERSITY

1. Admission consideration is offered only to those current matriculates in an AMA accredited veterinary curriculum, who believe that there are extenuating circumstances that would present significant hardship if they continue at their current institution.
2. Applicants requesting a transfer must contact the Dean of Academic and Student Success at the school they are currently attending and notify him or her of their intent.
3. Applicants must also demonstrate quality academic performance throughout their professional school enrollment.
4. The curricula of the two schools must be sufficiently alike to allow a student to enter the second-year class without deficiencies in academic background.
5. All selection criteria for regular applicants apply to transfer applicants.
6. Priority is given to Michigan residents.
7. Space must be available.
8. International students requesting a transfer also must fulfill all requirements set forth in the International Student Admissions Policy.

MIDWESTERN UNIVERSITY

Transfer Students
Midwestern University CVM may accept transfer students from other accredited veterinary schools on a case-by-case basis. Students requesting a transfer must meet all the standard admissions requirements. The final decision will be determined by the Associate Dean for Academic Affairs and the Dean.

Advanced Standing
All requests for advanced standing by admitted or enrolled students are processed on a course-by-course basis by the Office of the Dean. A student must submit a letter to the Office of the Dean in which the student lists the course(s) in which he or she is requesting advanced standing. The student must provide an official course description(s), a transcript, and a syllabus (syllabi) of the course(s) previously taken. All requests must be submitted prior to the start of the course being considered. The recommendation to grant or deny advanced standing will be made by the Dean in consultation with the department. It is expected that a minimum grade equal to a "B" would have been achieved in the class being petitioned.

UNIVERSITY OF MINNESOTA

1. Transfer students are accepted on a space available basis. The Admissions Committee will place each applicant in the year or semester of the curriculum deemed appropriate after analysis of equivalency of the required courses involved.
2. No academic work or standing will be accepted from DVM curricula other than those deemed accredited by the American Veterinary Medical Association.
3. All applicants must be U.S. citizens or holders of appropriate visas.
4. All applicants are required to have finished at least one full academic year at the institution from which transfer is requested and must be in good academic standing at the time of discontinuance according to written verification from the institution.
5. All applicants must have achieved a cumulative GPA of 3.00 (of 4.00) for the required courses at the initial institution.
6. Please visit the following website for more details: https://www.vetmed.umn.edu/education/dvm/transfer-students.

MISSISSIPPI STATE UNIVERSITY

The Mississippi State University College of Veterinary Medicine accepts, on a limited basis, transfer students from other veterinary medical colleges to fill vacancies in the freshmen or sophomore classes. Transfer guidelines are as follows:

From a veterinary school not accredited by the AVMA:

Applicants for transfer into the second semester of the first year must have completed coursework equivalent to coursework taught in the first semester of the first year at MSU-CVM.

Applicants for transfer into the first semester of the second year must have completed coursework equivalent to coursework taught in the first year at MSU-CVM.

Applicants for transfer into the second semester of the second year must have completed coursework equivalent to all coursework taught in the first three semesters at MSU-CVM plus have had equivalent surgery laboratories.

From a veterinary school accredited by the AVMA:

Applicants are considered on a case-by-case basis with regard to length of time in current program.

General:

Any applicant considered for transfer admission must be in good academic standing (defined as being eligible to continue at current school from current point in the curriculum), never have failed a course while in veterinary medical school, never have been dismissed from a veterinary school and must have completed at least a full academic year at current veterinary school.

An interview is required for any applicant considered for transfer admission. Interviews via Skype are acceptable.

Typically, transfer applicants are not accepted into our program at a point later than first semester of the sophomore year. Accordingly, if a student should pursue application to Mississippi State University College of Veterinary Medicine and be accepted, it would be necessary for that student to complete at least two years at Mississippi State University to be eligible for a degree.

Students accepted for transfer are required to meet the current computer requirements of the college.

For more information, contact Tonya Calmes, Admissions Assistant, 662-325-4161, tcalmes@cvm.msstate.edu.

UNIVERSITY OF MISSOURI

1. Must be a vacancy in the class.
2. Will consider students who are U.S. citizens or holders of permanent alien visas and who have finished at least two years in a college of veterinary medicine that is AVMA accredited.
3. Students must be in good academic standing, never been denied admission from the University of Missouri for a first year position, and submit a letter of reference from the dean's office of the present college is required.

NORTH CAROLINA STATE UNIVERSITY

Effective spring 2017, the NC State CVM no longer considers transfer application requests. Changes in our curriculum and the evolution of our DVM/PhD Program make this process change necessary.

THE OHIO STATE UNIVERSITY

Transfer students are considered. Each application is evaluated on an individual basis. For questions, please email cvm-dvmadmissions@osu.edu.

OKLAHOMA STATE UNIVERSITY

Transfer students are considered. Each application is evaluated on an individual basis. See website for transfer guide: http://www.cvhs.okstate.edu

OREGON STATE UNIVERSITY

Admission of students with advanced standing is considered only in certain circumstances, and each case is considered on an individual basis.

UNIVERSITY OF PENNSYLVANIA

Penn Vet considers transfer students, on an individual basis, for entry into the second year only (September). The availability of positions will be limited and the number of seats will not be known until approximately midsummer. The following requirements will be in effect:

1. Applicants will be required to have a minimum GPA of 3.00 without having repeated a course.
2. All Penn Vet prerequisite course requirements must be completed with a "C" or above before a transfer application may be submitted for consideration.
3. All major course work required by first-year students at Penn Vet must have been completed prior to matriculation. Missing material must be made up during the second academic year and must be completed prior to starting the third year.
4. Receipt of transcripts from all previously attended institutions, GRE scores and a letter of intent describing the reasons for wanting to transfer to Penn Vet. A copy of previous VMCAS application or a copy of application to current veterinary school.
4. Receipt of a letter from the Dean or Associate Dean of the home institution, indicating that the applicant is in good social and academic standing.

5. Application materials should be received by April 1. Be certain to include your email address to facilitate communication. For those who are finishing their first term in April, please have your transcripts sent as soon as possible. For other applicants, transcripts of previous terms should be available.

6. Send all materials to: Mary Bryant, VMD - Education & Student Affairs, The School of Veterinary Medicine, University of Pennsylvania, Rosenthal Building, 3800 Spruce Street, Philadelphia PA 19104

7. Interviews will be required and will be held during the applicant's spring break, usually in April if the applicant is in an on-going program. Those applicants who have a normal summer break may choose to interview early in that period.

Curricula vary among veterinary schools. Those coming from the most similar course work will be the most likely approved for transfer.

PURDUE UNIVERSITY

1. Positions must be available in the relevant class.
2. Student must be in good academic standing in his/her present program.
3. Students must have completed 1–2 years of DVM courses with an **exceptional** academic record in those courses.
4. Veterinary medical curricula must be compatible.
5. Student must have support of the administration from the program in which he/she is currently enrolled.

For more information, please email vetadmissions@purdue.edu.

UNIVERSITY OF TENNESSEE

Admission of students with advanced standing (transfer) may be considered for unique circumstances on a case-by-case basis.

1. Position(s) must be available in the class into which one would like to matriculate.
2. Curricula of the two schools must be sufficiently alike to allow a student to matriculate without deficiencies in his/her academic background.
3. The applicant's academic dean must provide a letter approving transfer and indicating that the student is in good standing at his/her current college/school of veterinary medicine.
4. Admission is usually limited to the second semester of the first year of the DVM curriculum except for exceptional circumstances.
5. Letters of reference are required.

The Admissions Committee will review applicant credentials and interview those determined to best meet admission criteria.

TEXAS A&M UNIVERSITY

Students requesting advanced standing must meet the following requirements:

1. Must have completed all previous professional veterinary courses in an AVMA accredited college of veterinary medicine.
2. Must have successfully completed the academic term preceding the semester into which student requests admission.
3. Must comply with all requirements for transfer into the university as described in the current catalog.
4. May request transfer only into the second through seventh semesters of the professional curriculum.
5. At the time of matriculation the student must certify by letter that he/she has not been convicted of crimes in the period from first enrollment in the college of veterinary medicine from which the student desires transfer until date of matriculation at Texas A&M University.
6. To request transfer consideration, the student must meet all requirements as posted on the College website at http://vetmed.tamu.edu/dvm/future/transferring.

TUFTS UNIVERSITY

Applicants from other veterinary schools are considered. Students with advanced standing are admitted if and when space becomes available in the second-year class. The application deadline is June 1 for the following September. Please refer to our website for details: http://vet.tufts.edu

TUSKEGEE UNIVERSITY

Tuskegee University College of Veterinary Medicine has a Non-Transfer Policy with other Veterinary Schools.

WASHINGTON STATE UNIVERSITY

Admission of students with advanced standing is considered only in very specific and unique circumstances, and each case is considered on an individual basis.

UNIVERSITY OF WISCONSIN

Wisconsin does not accept advanced standing students for admission.

INTERNATIONAL

ATLANTIC VETERINARY COLLEGE AT THE UNIVERSITY OF PRINCE EDWARD ISLAND

Applicants who have completed all or portions of a veterinary medical program may apply for advanced standing to the second year of the DVM program.

Applicants for advanced standing must present evidence of educational accomplishments and may be required to address missing courses or competencies expected of our incoming second-year students. Students admitted with advanced standing must begin the college year in September.

The candidate must file a formal application and may be interviewed by the Admissions Committee and possibly other faculty. Places for admission to the college with advanced standing are limited and depend on vacancies.

It is imperative that the Admissions Committee have detailed and translated summaries of veterinary medical academic programs and accomplishments for those seeking advanced placement from schools in foreign countries.

Advanced-standing applications should be on file and completed as early as possible and no later than January 1. Candidates are strongly encouraged to visit the website http://stage.upei.ca/avcpolicies/files/avcpolicies/avcaa_adm0004.pdf.

MASSEY UNIVERSITY

Applications for admission with advanced standing will only be considered by students enrolled in a veterinary program with a compatible curriculum, and pending an available space in the appropriate stage of the program. Applicants should contact vetschool@massey.ac.nz to apply for advanced standing.

MURDOCH UNIVERSITY

Applications for advanced standing will only be considered from students whose studies have been completed in a DVM program. Applicants are required to apply formally for advanced standing and provide the necessary documentation to allow for a full comparison between the previous study and Murdoch University's unit requirements. Prior courses must duplicate or substantially overlap multiple factors including breadth and depth of content, duration, objectives, assessment, context, and academic standard (level of intellectual effort required) for exemption to be granted.

ST. MATTHEW'S UNIVERSITY

Applications for admission with advanced standing are welcomed from students from veterinary schools recognized by the American Veterinary Medical Association (AVMA) and/or the American Association of Veterinary State Boards (AAVSB). Transfer applicants must submit a complete application package to ensure a timely review. Acceptance of transfer credit is at the discretion of St. Matthew's University.

UNIVERSITY OF CALGARY

Applications for admission to advanced semesters may be considered from students who have been enrolled in DVM programs at other institutions, subject to the availability of spaces in the DVM Program and the academic standing of the candidate. When places are available, candidates may be asked to present themselves for an interview and may be asked to pass examinations on subject matter in the veterinary curriculum. Applicants are advised that vacancies are rare and that restrictions on residency and citizenship status may be applied.

UNIVERSITÉ DE MONTRÉAL

1. Transfer students will only be considered for the beginning of the second year of veterinary medicine and only if transfer seats become available in that class.
2. Applicant must be enrolled in an AVMA-accredited college.
3. The applicant must have completed veterinary course work equivalent to that expected of the students in the DVM program of the Faculté de médecine vétérinaire de l'Université de Montréal, who will be in the second-year class.
4. Applicant must be a Canadian citizen or a permanent resident.
5. Applicant must fulfill the admission process as first-year students do.
6. Applicant shall contact the associate dean of studies of the FMV.
7. Applicant must complete the CASPER test.
8. Applicants who are not fluent in French must have a score of 785/990 at the TFI.

ROSS UNIVERSITY SCHOOL OF VETERINARY MEDICINE

Students who have completed a portion of the curriculum at another approved school of veterinary medicine may apply for admission with advanced standing. Such transfer applicants must present evidence of completion of courses (or their equivalent) at a school of veterinary medicine accredited by the American Veterinary Medical Association (AVMA), comparable to those offered in the pre-clinical curriculum of Ross University

School of Veterinary Medicine. Additionally, transfer students must meet all the requirements for admission.

Placement is determined by the Academic Promotions Committee and the Dean, and will depend on the courses already completed. Credit will not, however, be given for more than the first four semesters of study. Transfer students must take all of the courses offered for the semester they are admitted and may be required to repeat part or all of the curriculum.

THE UNIVERSITY OF QUEENSLAND

Applications for advanced standing will only be considered from students whose studies have been completed in a veterinary program with a compatible curriculum, and where a space is available in the appropriate stage of the program. Please refer to the University of Queensland Policy 3.50.03 - Credit for Previous Studies and Recognised Prior Learning (http://ppl.app.uq.edu.au) or contact the School directly (vetenquiries@uq.edu.au).

FIRST-YEAR PROFILE: AARON OLDANIE

Current School Name
Mississippi State University

Why do you want to be a veterinarian?
Veterinary medicine unites two of my favorite things: science and medicine. Every case is a mystery, and information from many subject areas must be incorporated to diagnose and treat the patient appropriately and effectively. Fostering the human-animal bond is also very important to me, not only from the emotional perspective, but also from a one-health perspective.

What are your short-term and long-term goals?
My current short-term goals as a veterinary student are to do my best in the DVM curriculum and decipher my specific interests in vet med. I also plan to get as much hands-on clinical/surgery experience this summer before our second-year surgery lab. Regarding my long-term goals, I plan to go into small animal medicine and possibly complete a surgery or internal medicine residency.

What did you do as an applicant to prepare for applying to veterinary school?
In my sophomore year of my undergraduate studies, I called as many veterinary offices in my area as I could. I started to volunteer at three of them. One of the clinics offered to hire and train me to be a veterinary assistant. On my days off, I started to volunteer at a large animal referral center to diversify my veterinary experiences. Academically, I took summer classes and graduated in three years, making sure to satisfy all of the prerequisites for the schools I was interested in attending.

What advice would you give to applicants or those considering applying to veterinary school?
It is very important to work hard and not give up on your dream. There are going to be a lot of volunteer and study hours, but it will all be worth it in the end. Staying focused is essential as well. Everything you do needs to be related to achieving your goal. It is not going to be easy, but if you want something bad enough, nothing can stop you. It is also never too late to start getting experience and to save your GPA if you work hard enough.

What helped make the transition to veterinary school easier for you?
Making friends early in veterinary school was helpful for me to transition. Our class is very supportive of one another. My undergraduate university also prepared me for the demanding curriculum of veterinary school. I enjoy exercising and doing outdoor activities. It is very easy to stay inside day in and day out to study, but it is important to take breaks and do something recreational.

What is your advice on student debt?
It is very easy to get overwhelmed with the amount of debt vet students accrue over a four-year program. Taking advantage of your university's financial planning tools is essential to keep finances organized. Living below your means is a big part of saving money. This doesn't mean starving yourself or living under an overpass, but rather doing little things like making food or coffee rather than eating out. Every little bit counts when you are spending borrowed money. In the end, the degree is worth much more than we pay to get it.

What are you most excited about learning in veterinary school?
I am most excited to learn surgery. I think it is an essential skill for veterinarians. I am excited to learn routine spay and neuter procedures that are important in population control measures. Soft tissue surgery and orthopedic surgeries also interest me because of the difference surgeons can make in the quality of life of the patient.

First Year Enrollment by Residency Status
at US Colleges of Veterinary Medicine
Internal AAVMC Data Reports
2017-2018

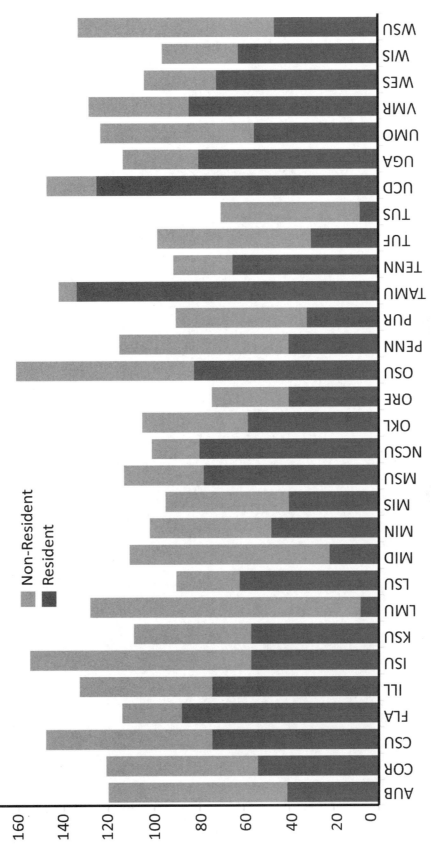

This visualization depicts enrollment by residency status for first year DVM students. Several US colleges of veterinary medicine allow DVM students to establish residency during the first year of matriculation; the change in residency status allows these students to pay resident tuition during their remaining three years in the professional program.

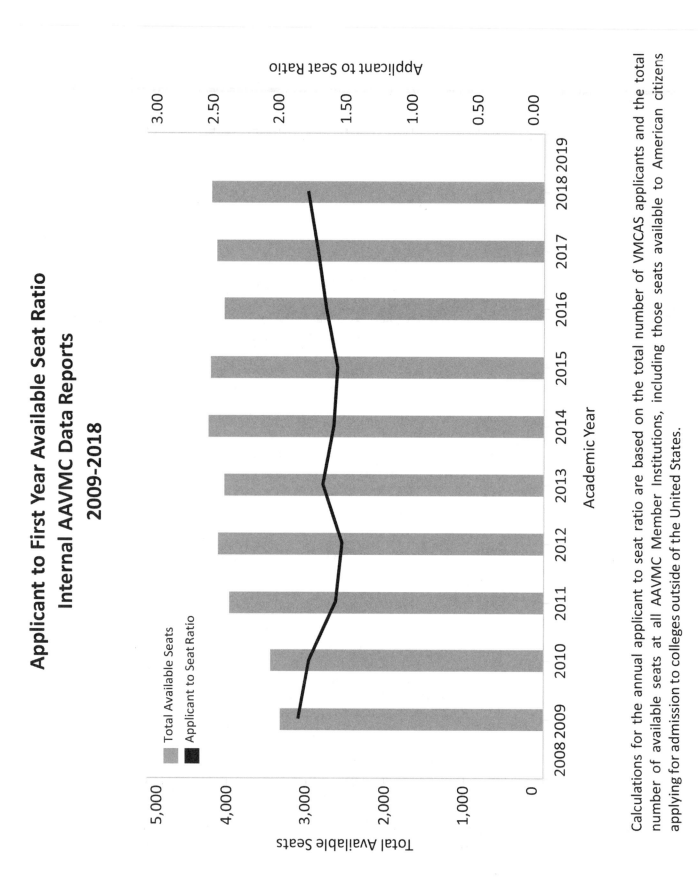

Applicant to First Year Available Seat Ratio
Internal AAVMC Data Reports
2009-2018

Total Available Seats

Applicant to Seat Ratio

Academic Year

Total Available Seats

Applicant to Seat Ratio

Calculations for the annual applicant to seat ratio are based on the total number of VMCAS applicants and the total number of available seats at all AAVMC Member Institutions, including those seats available to American citizens applying for admission to colleges outside of the United States.

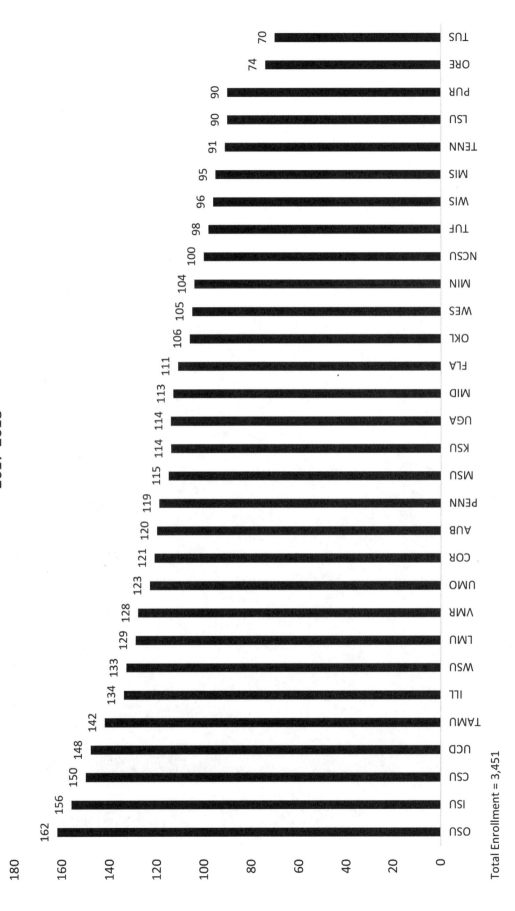

Number of Seats in the First-Year Class

By US College of Veterinary Medicine

AAVMC Internal Data Reports

2017-2018

Total Enrollment = 3,451

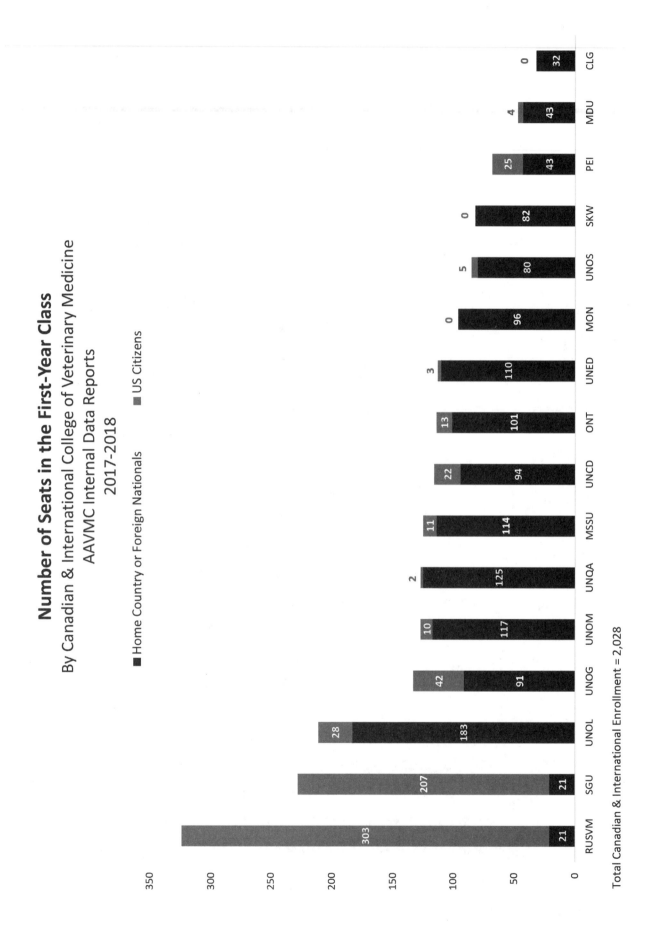

Number of Seats in the First-Year Class

By Canadian & International College of Veterinary Medicine

AAVMC Internal Data Reports

2017-2018

■ Home Country or Foreign Nationals ■ US Citizens

Total Canadian & International Enrollment = 2,028

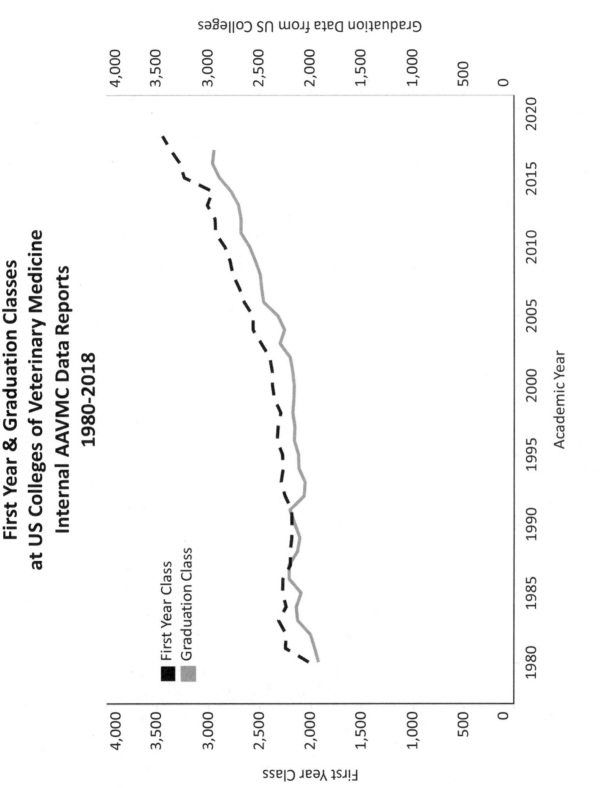

First Year & Graduation Classes
at US Colleges of Veterinary Medicine
Internal AAVMC Data Reports
1980-2018

Although the relationship between first year seats and graduation is expected to be a direct one, there are numerous reasons that explain perceived lags in graduation of DVM students. Numerous dual-degree options allow DVM students to step in and out of the professional curriculum.

First Year Enrollment by Residency Status
at US Colleges of Veterinary Medicine
Internal AAVMC Data Reports
2017-2018

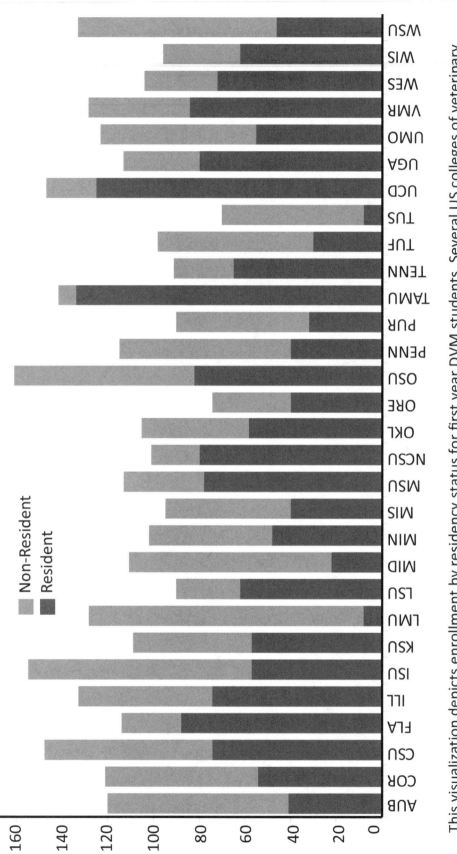

This visualization depicts enrollment by residency status for first year DVM students. Several US colleges of veterinary medicine allow DVM students to establish residency during the first year of matriculation; the change in residency status allows these students to pay resident tuition during their remaining three years in the professional program.